D1563166

WELL-BEING

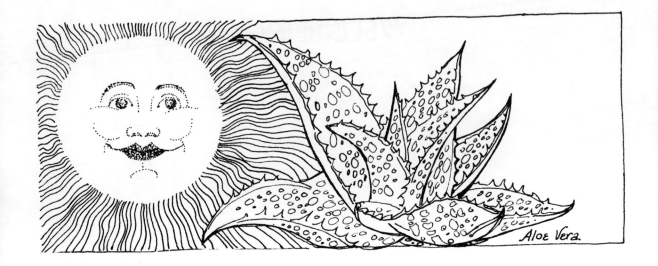
Aloe Vera.

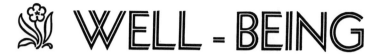

WELL - BEING

Edited by Barbara Salat
and David Copperfield

ANCHOR BOOKS
Anchor Press/Doubleday
Garden City, New York
1979

Contributors to WELL-BEING

edited by:
Barbara Salat, with the help of
David Copperfield
Allan Jaklich
Dean Plummer

written by:
Barbara Salat
Denni McCarthy
William LeSassier
David Copperfield
Kathi Keville
Rosemary Gladstar
Allan Jaklich
Jerrian J. Taber
Laura Burns
Michele Bigler

Suza Norton
Larry Wilson, M.D.
Larry and Sandy Shaw
Karen Shultz
Jim Hall, D.D.S.
David Debus
Elizabeth Spas
Michael Blate
Marianne Seidel
Harriet Korngold
Rita
Ginny Clark
John Bigler
Carole Johnson

art and photos by:
Jim Coit

Doug Kessing
Allan Jaklich
Christine Macy
Carole Johnson
Dean Plummer
Kathi Mignosi
Linda Luisi
Barbara Moody
Melanie Nielson
Michele Bigler
Steve Jeffres
Roslie Kessing
Louise
Katie McGee
Harriet Korngold
Juliette Mondot

The Anchor Books edition is the first publication of WELL-BEING in book form.
Anchor Books edition: 1979

Library of Congress Cataloging in Publication Data
Main entry under title:

Well-being.

A selection of articles from Well-Being magazine.
Includes index.
1. Naturopathy. 2. Herbs—Therapeutic use.
3. Health. I. Salat, Barbara. II. Copperfield, David.
RZ440.W44   615′.882
ISBN: 0-385-14221-8
Library of Congress Catalog Card Number 78–1219

CONTENTS

INTRODUCTION

Here is a book about twentieth-century folk medicine. It is written by modern pioneers: back-to-the-landers, gardeners, teachers, cooks, doctors, midwives, mothers, and just plain people. It is not intended to be the last word on natural health or well-being, but it is perhaps a good reflection on the state of the art of home remedies and self-treatment.

Today, people are concerned about learning how to take care of themselves and how to live well simply. The articles in WELL-BEING are all taken from personal experiences and are easy for anyone to understand and apply. Although we feel confident of their accuracy and honesty, we urge each person to judge the material for him or her self. Each person is different, and may respond differently to natural methods. They are safe methods, though, and lend themselves to experimentation or "practice," if you will.

We recommend that newcomers to this material begin with the preventive techniques and treatment of simple disorders. That's the way we most easily learn. We've stuck to usable material on herbs, knowing that although they have been used to treat successfully such disorders as arthritis, profuse hemorrhaging, etc., most people aren't prepared to deal with these complex conditions without professional help. We've tried wherever we can to bring scientific and lay understandings together to complement each other.

There will always be controversy and disagreement in the scientific world. This is part of its nature. Folk medicine, on the other hand, has always been based on "what works," because people need that sort of down-to-earth information. The modern folk medicine is not based on superstition, and tries to learn from its professional counterpart. We see this as a positive attitude which can benefit both worlds. We hope you will enjoy this volume, and that it will be good for your well-being.

If you enjoy our book you may want to read our magazine. All the material here was taken from articles in the monthly magazine *Well-Being*. The magazine continues to report on the latest and best that twentieth-century folk medicine has to offer. For further information, write to *Well-Being,* P. O. Box 1829, Santa Cruz, California 95061.

WELL-BEING

HOW'S YOUR HEALTH?

by Larry Wilson, M.D.

WAYS OF DIAGNOSING HEALTH

We hear a lot about diagnosing illness. What about diagnosing health? Is health simply the absence of disease? Or is there a positive state of health that we can detect in ourselves?

Edward Carpenter in his essay "Civilization, Its Cause and Cure" reminds us that the word health is derived from the same root as the words holy, hale, whole, and wholesome. Health, he says, is a condition of unity of body, mind, and spirit—all functioning together as one. Disease is the breakup of that unity, the establishment of subordinate centers or foci: infections, tumors, or neuroses. As there are many ways to break up a unity, so there are hundreds of diseases.

Similarly, oriental medicine describes health as the harmonious flow of vital energy through the body, while illness is a disordering or diversion of the flow—too little to one organ, too much to another. Alexis Carrel, in his excellent book, *Man, the Unknown,* defines true health, as opposed to artificial or false health. Artificial health is that which modern medicine affords us—we seem well, but need the constant attention of doctors, hospitals, pills, and operations to stay well. Natural or true health, he says, is the state in which we aren't dependent on an army of professionals—the body has the power to resist infestations and infections on its own. It is the condition in which we find so-called primitive peoples and wild animals in their natural environment—and is the condition that all people really desire.

We can synthesize the above and say that health is a state of wholeness, of unity and harmony of the body with its parts, which results in a natural immunity or resistance to disease.

But what are the signs and symptoms of positive health? How can we tell our own condition?

A good place to start is with the signs of good digestion—without good digestion there can't be good health. If we examine our stools, are they dark brown, blackish, light brown, or bronze-colored? They ought to be bronze-colored. Are they malodorous? They ought not be. Bad odor or dark color indicates that our food is not digesting properly—that a certain amount is rotting or fermenting, generating poisonous substances and not nourishing us at all. Gas, belching, a coated tongue, and poor appetite are further signs of poor digestion. Finally, many people have sluggish bowels, or constipation. We ought to go to the toilet twice a day, or after each big meal. Once a day, or once every two days, is not enough if we are eating the usual quantity of food.

Another set of signs are those we observe when the body contains waste matter that can't be handled by the normal eliminative channels, and therefore seeks other outlets. The common signs are bad breath—an elimination through the lungs, and poor complexion—an abnormal elimination through the skin. As health improves, the breath becomes sweet, the skin smooth and clear, and dandruff will disappear; the monthly discharge of menstrual blood will also lessen, though this has no relation to lowered fertility.

Our state of health is also indicated by certain psychological and mental signs and symptoms. If we find ourselves constantly fatigued, or unable to sleep well, or dominated by anger, fears, hatreds, or envy, we have a way to go to achieve health. Poise, a calm disposition, faith, cheerfulness, a loving attitude, gratitude, a sense of wonder, desire to be active, and positiveness are signs of health, and in themselves are powerful healing forces.

Recognizing the above signs will tell you much more than a doctor's yearly checkup. You can know more about your own condition than any doctor. When we ignore or suppress the above signs, we open the way for illness. Every heart at-

tack, stroke, ulcer, tumor, or infection is preceded by some of the signs of poor health that we've mentioned.

Signs and Symptoms of Health

good	poor
Sweet breath.	Bad breath.
Clear tongue.	Coated tongue.
Good appetite.	Poor appetite.
Clear complexion.	Skin eruptions/pimples, dandruff.
Stools well formed, bronze-colored, without bad odor.	Stools very light to dark brown or blackish, with bad odor.
Energy and desire to be active.	Fatigue.
Undisturbed sleep.	Difficult sleep.
Poise, calm disposition.	Tension, nervousness.
Cheerfulness, confidence, gratitude.	Anger, fears, distrust, envy.
Positive attitude.	Negative attitude.

THE BASICS OF HEALTH IMPROVEMENT

We are offered a hundred ways to become healthier, from medicine and surgery to acupuncture, diets, fasting, chiropractic, psychotherapy, herbs, etc. How do we find our way through all this?

The above methods or treatments may be useful in a particular person and condition, and each deserves a separate discussion. However, the *basis* for positive health is not to be found in any of these.

If we truly desire well-being, we need to concentrate our efforts in the more mundane realm of our daily living habits, or hygiene. It is these habits, taken together, that determine our health more than anything else. "Treatments" can be useful, but their effects are often not lasting. If we return to bad habits, the problem will recur.

Our habits include what, when, and how much we eat, how much we sleep and exercise, the quality of the air we breathe and water we drink, the work we do, where we live, the people we surround ourselves with, and the psychological atmosphere we place ourselves in. Improving our health is mainly a matter of modifying our bad habits, ordering our lives—taking control.

Changing old habits requires discipline and patience with ourselves; but if the goal is kept in mind, the changes will come. I don't know of any shortcuts, and the process takes months and years to accomplish in some people. I look at it as a challenge—something to have fun with. If it is seen as a giant sacrifice or duty, this is sure to cause more problems than it may alleviate. I view it as an experiment in good living, and find that the benefits far outweigh the inconveniences. I encourage folks to try modifying their habits, but not to force it.

The study of correct living habits—or how we were designed to live—is called hygiene science. There are excellent books available by Dr. Herbert Shelton, Dr. John Tilden, Norman Walker, Jethro Kloss, and others. I'll summarize some of their conclusions:

On the matter of eating—our food needs to be "natural," grown without synthetic fertilizers or pesticides, and eaten as much as possible in its natural state, with a predominance of fresh fruits, vegetables, nuts, and seeds. We need to avoid processed and artificial foods, additives whose effects are not well known, bad food combinations, and any foods that we don't digest well. Most folks need to eat less and observe good eating habits. Avoid: drinking with meals, eating without true hunger, eating when upset or tired, eating before going to bed. Eat slowly and chew thoroughly. Eat in a quiet, relaxed place, with good company, and discuss only pleasant topics during meals. It is also excellent to rest a few minutes after eating, rather than dashing away from the table.

The body must also have adequate exercise, as well as enough rest and sleep. Many people are chronically tired. We need fresh air twenty-four hours per day, and pure water (free of chlorine, fluorine, and other chemicals). We ought to live in a tranquil, secure, attractive place surrounded by people who enable us to relax and be ourselves. Boisterous or aggressive people can be as poisonous as arsenic. Our mental diet—TV, radio, movies, papers, magazines, books—also needs to be monitored and ordered to avoid pollution of the mind with false ideas or silly preoccupations.

Upon adopting a healthy regimen, the signs of health will begin to appear. No one is ever too old or too sick to begin.

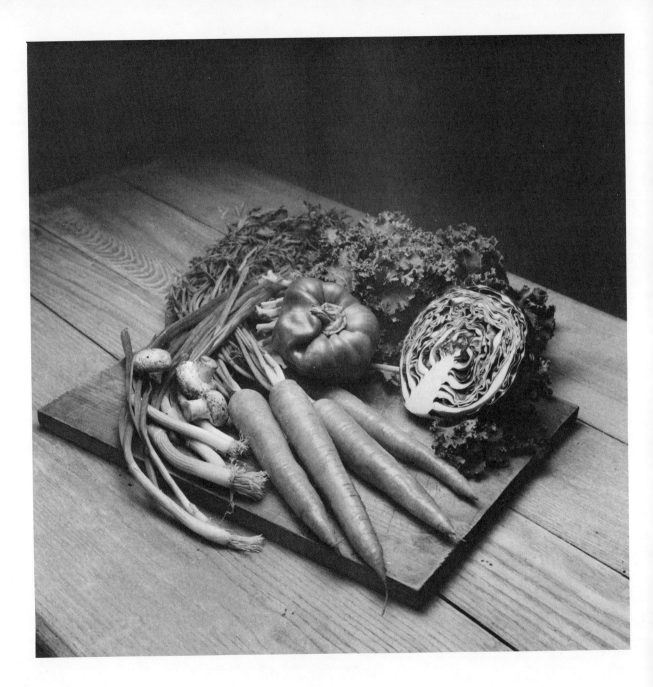

I

HEALTHFUL DIETS PAST AND PRESENT

HEALTHFUL DIETS PAST AND PRESENT

by Suza Norton

What is a good natural diet? There is no single "best" diet, but there are many native dietary patterns which, if understood and applied, will provide high-quality nutrition. The primitive people recorded in Dr. Weston Price's book *Nutrition and Physical Degeneration* had virtually perfect teeth and superb skeletal structure. Their particular native dietaries were selected in accordance with the accumulated wisdom of their race. Let's look at a few of the common denominators found among those primitive diets analyzed by Dr. Price.

1. *All foods were grown in highly mineralized soils* with considerable humus content, and without poisonous sprays, etc.

2. *They ate whole foods, not fractionalized parts of foods.* They did not remove by refining, or otherwise, the valuable fiber, vitamin, and mineral content of their natural foods.

3. In each diet plan, among those healthy primitives studied all over the world, *there was some source of unaltered, raw protein* (especially important during pregnancy). For us, this source could be sprouted seeds, raw milk products, fresh raw seeds and nuts, fertile, ground-fed eggs—raw or prepared at low heat—or meat cooked at low temperatures.

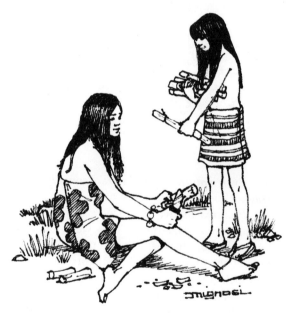

4. (In Dr. Price's words) "In general all the native foods were found to contain two to six times as high a factor of safety in the matter of *body building minerals* as did the displacing (refined) foods."

5. *Minerals, fat-soluble vitamins, and activator "X"* from high-vitamin butter and cream, seafoods, cod liver oil, seal oil, and animal organs with their fats were consumed by nearly all

groups studied. Use real raw butter instead of margarine. Drink whole raw milk, not low-fat pasteurized milk.

6. *Some sort of sea plant or animal was a part of every diet.* Inland sea deposits were treasured and used thriftily. Use kelp and dulse especially if a vegetarian.

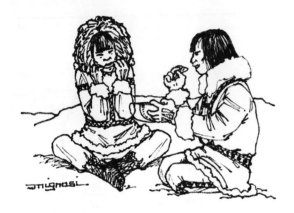

7. *Even natural sweets were generally used sparingly.*

8. *Primitive native foods were all abundant in the nitrilosides* (laetriles). They were found in the passion fruit in the tropics, the millet and sprouts of the Orient, and the apricots and other fruits which were eaten with their kernels. Cattle and other animals ate nitriloside-rich grasses, and their butter, milk, cheese, cream, and tissues contained this protective food factor.

9. The only methods of food preservation and storage that were used were those which *altered the nutrients the least amount:* earth storage, drying, freezing in cold climates, or those methods which made the nutrients in foods more

available such as culturing, pickling, fermenting, and sprouting.

10. *Generally, all foods were eaten raw or gently cooked,* or prepared in a manner which kept the nutrients intact.

11. Also very important, each healthy primitive group *observed regular periods of undereating, fasting, or partial abstinence from food,* either through naturally imposed food-limiting factors, rituals, or taboos. A person who reaches forty, and who has not regularly practiced at least semi-fasting, should introduce this practice gradually to his body, and realize that often he or she has many days to make up for. Make a study of body-cleansing diets to find one that is suitable for you.

12. *Children were breast-fed for generally two to three years.* Most people had means for spacing children at least two to three years apart, to protect the health of both mother and child.

13. At the time of Dr. Price's study, *all people studied had access to pure water, sunlight, and air,* important for health both of plants (which we eat) and people. And naturally, the *lifestyle was active and out of doors* as much as the climate allowed.

In essence, the people Dr. Price studied that were in good health understood fully the last and most important statement in his book, that, "Life in all its fullness, is Mother Nature obeyed."

The Price-Pottenger Foundation is carrying on the research and educational work of Dr. Price. For membership information and a list of publications, write to P. O. Box 2614, La Mesa, California 92041.

QUICK FOODS: NUTRITION ON THE GO

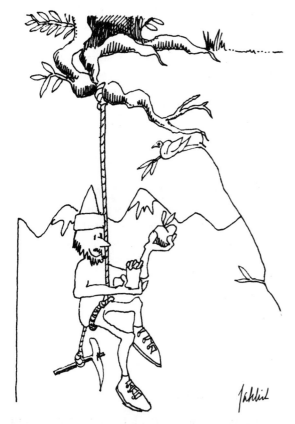

Everyone's in a hurry! Although we should take our time preparing food, many of us don't have the time. If canned, frozen, dried, processed, "convenience" foods turn you off, consider these natural foods alternatives.

FOODS TO KEEP ON HAND

Buckwheat groats—need only to be steeped or lightly cooked. They are good for breakfast, lunch (mix with herbs and veggies and flour for bucky burgers), or stuffed in cabbage leaves for a quick, special dinner.

Tofu—a quick to fix, easily digested protein food. It can be used for breakfast (scrambled), sautéed in tamari for a tofu sandwich, used in vegetable dishes or as a base for a creamy salad dressing. See *The Book of Tofu* for more suggestions.

Tortillas—(the corn-flour kind with no preservatives) warmed over the burner of a stove and served with raw or steamed veggies, cheese, or avocados, make an easy, satisfying meal.

Cashews—good gravy! (see recipe page 11) A good addition to salads, desserts, or main dishes.

Curry—can make any vegetable dish or soup special.

Miso—a substitute for soup stock or bouillon. With a little brewer's yeast, makes a beefy broth. Adds flavor and nutrition to soups, loafs, spreads, and other dishes.

Sprouts—good with any meal or as a snack for quick energy.

Noodles—hearty, quick addition to soups, vegetable dishes, or just serve plain with a sauce.

There are many kinds of wholesome noodles: spinach, buckwheat, sesame, artichoke, egg, and others.

Fruits—are good for a snack or a meal, except after eating grains or beans.

THINGS TO MAKE AHEAD

Salad dressing—make your favorites in large enough quantities to last a few days, or all week.

Herb vinegar—add your favorite salad herbs, and perhaps a clove of garlic to a bottle of apple cider vinegar. Shake daily, and you will have a valuable last-minute salad dressing; just add olive oil and water, or a tomato and mayonnaise.

Soy loaf—if your family likes heavy protein meals, make enough of your favorite loaf to keep on hand all week for quick-to-fix soy patties, to warm up with eggs in the morning (soy sausages), to make a last-minute meatloaf, or to blend up with water, adding diced vegetables, to make a cream of soy soup. Every once in a while our family gets hungry for soybeans. It saves a lot of preparation time to keep this mix on hand.

Frozen bananas—choose fairly ripe, but still firm, bananas, peel them, put them in a plastic bag and freeze them; for making smoothies nothing is better. Also if you have a juicer, they make a delicious ice cream-like non-dairy dessert; just run them through. (For Champion or Norwalk type juicers only.)

Herb tea—make enough beverage or medicinal tea to last all day. Refrigerate in a closed container. Reheat gently.

Nut and seed butter—grind sesame, sunflower, or pumpkin seeds, almonds, or cashews in a nut grinder. Add a small amount of light, high-quality oil to make a butter. The butters may be mixed together. Peanut and almond butter is especially good as a sandwich spread or as a base for candies. Just mix with honey and roll in coconut. Remember to buy in bulk nuts that are untreated for the best in nutrition and price.

SOME HINTS:

1. When you are in a rush and can't even sit down for a meal, a smoothy is a good solution to your hunger problem. But remember, sip, don't gulp.

2. Making a quick scan of your cabinets and refrigerators can spark your imagination. Be creative with what is on hand. Raw vegetables and a dip are often a satisfying, light, quick meal.

3. Especially if you are tense, take thirty seconds to relax, breathe deeply, and give thanks for your food; you will be glad you did.

RAW APPLE SAUCE

Chop 2 apples. Put through a food grinder or blend with 2 tablespoons of any kind of pure fruit juice, adding honey or cinnamon if desired.

TOFU CHILIQUILES

1 green pepper
½ medium onion
oil
½ cup water
2 teaspoons chili powder
½ pound tofu
cayenne (optional)

Chop pepper into large bite-sized pieces. Chop onion into smaller pieces. Sauté in small amount of good oil. Add water, chili powder, and tofu which has been cut up into bite-sized chunks. Simmer 5 minutes, serve. Cheese may also be added. Good in tortillas.

QUICK BIRTHDAY CAKE

4 cups flour
1 tablespoon baking powder
1 teaspoon salt
2 cups honey
½ cup butter
½ cup oil
½ cup water (juice or milk)
3 eggs
2 teaspoons vanilla or almond extract

Combine dry ingredients. Add to wet ingredients. Bake at 350° for 30–35 minutes. Frost with whipped cream. (Please do not use baking powder that contains aluminum.)

CASHEW MILK

1 cup nuts
3½ cups water

Blend. Enjoy on cereals, in baking, with pero (coffee substitute), or with honey (1–2 teaspoons per cup). Keep refrigerated.

CASHEW GRAVY (White Sauce)

2 cups cashew milk
¾ cup cold water
1 tablespoon arrowroot powder

Warm the cashew milk. Mix water and arrowroot powder. Add to milk. Simmer 10 minutes. Stir occasionally as it thickens. Use as it is, or add any seasonings. A good basic gravy or sauce.

QUICK VEGETABLE DRINK

1 large tomato
a few celery leaves
some green peppers, watercress, green onions,
    parsley, or whatever
a bit of lemon juice

Blend.

BREAKFASTS WORTH GETTING UP FOR

There are so many ways to have breakfast. Here are menus and recipes for three different situations. Plan time for a good breakfast every morning. Even if you have only a cup of tea, the time you take will nourish you. All these meals are relatively quick and simple. Some can be prepared the night before if you're in a hurry in the morning.

MIXED FRUIT COCKTAIL
GREEK TOFU PIE
SOY SAUSAGES
SPROUTS

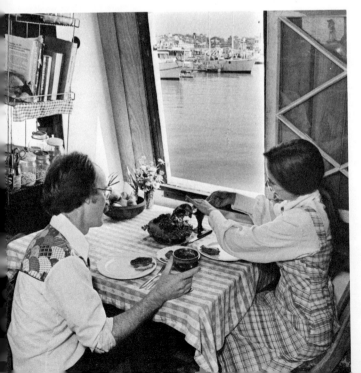

MIXED FRUIT COCKTAIL

Blend the juice of ½ grapefruit with 1 cup apricot juice. Add 4 sliced strawberries and 2 sliced apricots. Serves 2.

GREEK TOFU PIE

Press 1 cake tofu overnight and squeeze to remove excess moisture.

Add 1 tablespoon oregano
     1 tablespoon Bronner's Protein Seasoning
or lesser amount of saltier seasoning

Put this in a 9-inch whole-wheat pie crust, fold crust over the top, and press sides together on top, sealing.

Bake at 350° 30 minutes.

Serve on a plate of leafy buckwheat sprouts and garnish top with parsley. (It's good cold too.)

Serves 4.

SOY SAUSAGES

Use any soy burger or loaf recipe

Add extra flour if necessary to hold together.

Form into little "sausage" pieces and grill in a lightly oiled pan for about 10 minutes.

CREAM OF WHATEVER SOUP
TOAST OR CRACKERS
SPROUTS

FRUIT SALAD
YOGHURT
HERB TEA

CREAM OF WHATEVER SOUP

1 cup hot water
½ cup cashews
2 cups whatever: celery, onions, parsley,
    watercress, or other convenient veggies. Even
    leftover steamed vegetables will do. Chop,
    slice, or grate them into small pieces.
1 teaspoon salt
1 teaspoon oil

Blend until almost smooth, then add 2 cups hot water and heat, but don't boil. Garnish with sprouts.
Serves 2.

FRUIT SALAD

Combine in a large bowl

½ pineapple in chunks
1 basket strawberries, sliced
small handful of shredded coconut, toasted or
    raw
Brazil nuts
dash of cinnamon

Lace with honey to taste.
Arrange orange sections around the sides of the bowl and top with borage flowers if you have them.
Serves 4.

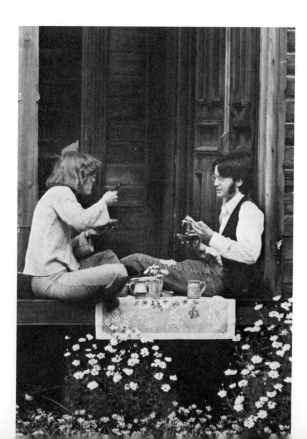

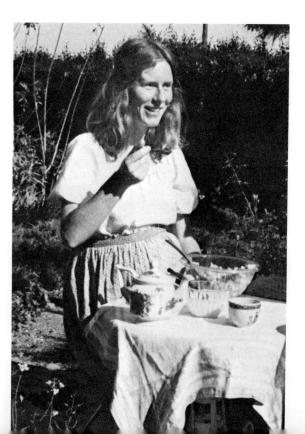

LUNCH BOX FOODS

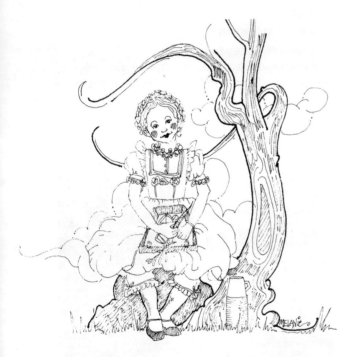

One of the problems nutrition-minded parents face is preparing adequate lunch-box meals for their children to eat at school. What a child will eat in his own home and what he will eat with his friends may be two different things. At home foods such as raw vegetables, fruit, and brown bread may seem natural. But at school, in the midst of hot dogs, pop, sugar this and sugar that, a child might feel his food is odd, and his friends might encourage him in this.

Here are a few suggestions to try if you find yourself in this situation:

1. First and always, communicate. Find out what's happening and why. Talk about what is most important to you and what is most important to your child.

2. Plan lunches together, and if possible, make them in the evening so there's plenty of time to enjoy being together and creative. Children often like the same thing day after day, which makes things easier.

3. If you are going to be different, remember to keep the lines of communication open between you and your child. This can be a great lesson for you, your child, and his schoolmates. Children (and some adults) sometimes put down anything that is different, but once the initial reaction wears off, the other kids don't get a charge from poking fun.

NUTRITIOUS ADDITIONS TO ANY LUNCH
bee pollen
celery with peanut butter or cream cheese
a tomato
dulse (beef jerky of the sea)
rice crackers

carrot chips (Raw carrots sliced very thinly on the broad blade of a grater. The best grater is a sauerkraut grater. It makes very thin slices which are easy to chew and juicy.)

a hard-steeped egg (Steeping, or coddling an egg is a much gentler way of cooking it than simmering or boiling. Just drop the egg into boiling water, cover the pot, and turn the heat off. Let it "steep" for 10–15 minutes. This makes a much more easily digested egg, and also saves on energy.)

OTHER HINTS

try making egg salad with tofu to cut down on eggs.

try slipping some raw vegetables into cheese sandwiches. They add a crunchy texture.

MEATLESS MEALS

Some people call this vegetarian chopped liver. What you call it depends on how you season it and who you're trying to fool. It involves no cooking, and is quick to fix and contains a good supply of protein. Use it on bread, chips, crackers, celery, or other vegetables. Experiment with various seasonings to suit your taste.

1 cup sunflower seeds
½ cup walnuts
1 dozen medium-sized mushrooms
1 stalk celery
3 scallions
1 small carrot
½ cup zucchini
1 tomato
dash of tamari
dash of oil
suggested seasonings:
   caraway
   chervil
   curry
   oregano
   thyme

To prepare:

Grind seeds and nuts in blender or nut grinder. Chop finely mushrooms, celery, and scallions. Grate finely carrot and zucchini. Liquefy tomato.

Mix all remaining ingredients, adding each to taste.

WALNUT CHEESE LOAF

2 cups (4 slices) bread crumbs
1½ cups grated cheese
1 cup milk
1 egg, beaten
1–1½ cups scarcely chopped walnuts
1–1½ cups chopped celery (optional)
1–1½ cups chopped mushrooms (optional)
2 tablespoons parsley and other spices
   (up to ¼ cup)
salt and pepper

Top with mushroom soup or yoghurt and mayonnaise blend.
Bake at 350° 30–40 minutes.

STUFFED SOY LOAF

Simmer, covered, for 1 hour:

1 cup soy grits
½ cup rice
3 cups water (You may need more. Keep an
   eye on it.)
oregano
basil
rosemary

Combine while grits cook:

1 onion, diced
1 pepper, diced
4 tablespoons miso
2 tablespoons oil
1 tomato, puréed
1 tablespoon salt

Mix grits and vegetables and add:
whole-wheat flour—just enough to make the loaf hold together

Stuffing
Combine:

¼ cup pumpkin seeds
¼ cup peanuts
2 cups bread crumbs
½ cup diced celery
2 tablespoons butter, softened
1 egg or a little milk or water
caraway
thyme
a little soy loaf mix

Put half of the loaf into an 8- or 9-inch glass pie pan. Put stuffing in center, then cover with rest of the loaf.

Bake at 300° 45 minutes to 1 hour until browned, a little crusty, but not too dry inside.

Whether you are a protein-conscious vegetarian or a meat eater who wishes to explore the alternatives, it is good to know how to prepare a variety of meatless meals. Let's face it, beans aren't beef, and if you expect a soyburger to taste like a hamburger you will be disappointed. Instead, if you complement the natural flavors of beans and grains with vegetables, herbs, and spices, you'll create distinctive, nutritious, inexpensive meals that you'll soon acquire a taste for. The following is a favorite recipe of mine:

SOYBURGERS

Simmer 1 hour (can be done ahead of time):
1 cup soy grits in
2 cups water

Combine thoroughly while grits cook:

some chopped onion
green pepper
celery
garlic
mushrooms
1 cup leftover rice or other grain
vegetable salt
thyme
oregano
basil

(Vary amounts of vegetables and herbs to taste.)

miso or soy sauce
¼ cup oil

Combine all ingredients, then add:
whole wheat flour
soy flour (optional)
egg (optional)

Use enough flour (and egg if you use it) to make a firm mixture; mixing thoroughly will develop gluten in the flour which will help it stick together.

Form into ¼-inch patties.

Fry in small amount of oil about 10–15 minutes.

Serve with your favorite "fixin's."

Store leftovers in refrigerator or freezer.

May be used for "meatloaf" or as "sausages" with eggs.

WARMING UP FOR WINTER

The aroma of fresh baked bread, of a simmering stew or a fresh pot of rice is in itself a thawing comfort to a chilly or wet soul. In winter we are generally less active. The following are suggestions for foods which will help warm you up on those chilly days.

Buckwheat
Said to be the most heat-generating of grains, this is a favorite in such famous cold spots as Siberia.

Curry powder*
This blend of spices varies greatly from mild, American flavored to barely bearable authentic Indian-style. Try a variety of brands or blend your own.* It lends its flavors to soups, rice,* vegetables, crackers, or salad dressings.

Ginger
Dried ginger is handy for a quick cup of tea, or to season fruit or vegetable dishes. Fresh ginger can be added, grated or diced, to grains or vegetables or can be easily pickled to eat as a side dish.*

Cayenne
An excellent warmer and seasoning. Use in sauces, soups, sprinkle on salads or other foods, and put a little in your socks if you have cold feet.

Chili powder
Varies widely in flavor. Try different brands, or dry peppers (blend sweet and hot) and grind

*means recipe follows.

them to make your own. Especially good to season tofu, beans, corn bread, or eggs. With most varieties there's no need to use sparingly.

Hot sauce
There are some brands of hot sauce which are chemical-free. You can also make your own.* It is a handy seasoning to keep on the table.

Yogi tea
A blend of warming spices that's good "straight" or with milk and honey. Can also be mixed with apple juice or juices of orange and lemon for a great punch that warms you all over. There are many different recipes and blends.*

Onion
Is commonly overlooked as a vegetable, being mostly used as a seasoning. Use red onion raw on salads. Bake or steam yellow onions.*

Garlic
Can be used and reused in many ways. Whole garlic cloves are delightful baked in their skins or served as a tasty condiment pickled in vinegar or vinegar and honey. Garlic butter is an all-around favorite. For real enthusiasts, make garlic soup. Parsley is a good antidote for garlic breath.

RECIPES

WARM MILK AND HONEY

Warm the milk slowly, please, adding honey to your taste. Add roasted carob or turmeric if so inclined. Pour in favorite ceramic mug and snuggle in best blanket. Drink!

HOT APPLE CIDER

Heat cider, adding cinnamon, cloves, nutmeg, and a pinch ginger (and if you like, some curry) according to taste and amount of cider. Pour in mugs with cinnamon sticks to stir and suck on.

YOGI TEA

    4 3-inch-long cinnamon sticks
    10 whole cloves
    1 small fresh ginger root or several small dried
        ones
    5 allspices
    10 cardamom seeds
    1 gallon water

Proportions vary widely, according to individual tastes. Simmer on very low heat for a long time, anywhere from ½ to 3 hours. Several servings of tea can be made from the same herbs.

GARLIC SPREAD

Blend till smooth:

    ¾ cup oil (part olive and soy)
    6–7 cloves fresh garlic
    1 tablespoon dry onion powder
    2 tablespoons chopped parsley
    ¼ teaspoon sea salt

SALSA (fresh, not cooked)

Chiles—Use small jalapeño chiles. (These chiles are quite warming—some might even call

them hot—so, when using canned or fresh ones, remember you can always add more if you want them, but they can't be removed once they are mixed in!)

Fresh chiles—Place the chiles on the grill or broil until the skin is burned. Turn them if need be so that all sides get done. Remove them and cover with a wet towel. Peel off the burned skin. Chop them very fine.

Canned chiles—Use a small can
    squirt of lemon
    green onions
    whole tomatoes (skins removed by setting
        them in a steamer for just a few minutes; the
        skins then come off easily)
    oregano
    oil
    garlic
    salt and pepper
    tomato sauce (½ small can, or use fresh
        stewed tomatoes)
    cilantro (coriander)

Mix all together; store in refrigerator. Will keep for one week.

CURRY POWDER

Grind together in a blender for at least five minutes:

    2 teaspoons coriander seeds (whole)
    ½ teaspoon cumin seeds (whole)
    2 cardamom seeds, cut in half
    2 whole cloves
    ½ teaspoon powdered mace
    ⅙ teaspoon powdered allspice
    1 bay leaf cut up very fine
    3 sprigs fresh thyme or ⅙ teaspoon dry
    1 teaspoon fenugreek seeds (whole)
    2 teaspoons powdered turmeric
    2 chiles, Japanese type

FRESH HORSERADISH

1 large horseradish root
1 cup white wine or wine vinegar (cider
     vinegar causes root to turn dark)

Remove skin, grate into vinegar, bottle, and
cork tightly. Maybe add a little salt.

LENTIL SOUP

2 cups lentils (wash please—no stones)
1 onion
1 tablespoon sea salt
2 cloves garlic, chopped
thyme and marjoram
pepper to taste
2 quarts water
3 nice-sized carrots (greens of one chopped
     fine)
2 stalks celery and greens
1 bunch spinach

Put lentils and herbs in water, bring to boil,
adding vegetables in order as you chop them
minus spinach. Simmer for a couple of hours.
Then cook for 10 minutes longer, add spinach for
last few minutes.

STEAMED ONION

Peel and quarter 1 large onion
Steam 10 minutes. Remove water.
Simmer 5 minutes more with:

1 teaspoon butter
½ teaspoon caraway seeds

Serve with applesauce and/or sauerkraut.

MISO BROTH

1 cup boiling water
Remove from heat.
1 tablespoon favorite miso
Stir in, let cool slightly. Drink!

GINGERBREAD

½ cup butter
¼ cup honey
¾ cup molasses
1 egg (optional)
1 cup raw milk
2½ cups whole-wheat flour
½ teaspoon salt
1 tablespoon freshly ground ginger
1 teaspoon each freshly ground cinnamon and
     nutmeg
1 teaspoon vanilla

Cream together butter, honey, and molasses.
Stir egg into milk, mix well, and slowly add to
creamed mixture. Gradually stir in flour, salt,
spices, and flavoring. Pour into a pan and pop it
in the oven. Bake about 45 minutes at 350°, or 3
hours in a solar oven. Yum! Whipped cream on
top is delicious.

BAKED RICE PUDDING

2 cups cooked brown rice
½ cup raisins
½ teaspoon grated lemon rind
1 teaspoon lemon juice
½ cup honey
¼ teaspoon sea salt
½ teaspoon vanilla
3 eggs
2½ cups milk

Preheat oven to 325°. Place rice, raisins, rind, and juice in a buttered 1½-quart baking dish. Beat together remaining ingredients and pour over rice and raisins. Stir to mix. Bake 30 minutes or till pudding is set. Serves 4.

CAROB CAROLING DRINK

2 teaspoons carob
½ teaspoon cinnamon (vary to taste)
⅛ teaspoon nutmeg (vary to taste)
2 teaspoons pero (optional)
2 tablespoons honey
1 teaspoon butter (optional)
¼ cup sesame seeds
1 teaspoon vanilla
1½ cups hot water

Toast seeds, grind in grinder or blender. Add other ingredients. Add water and blend.

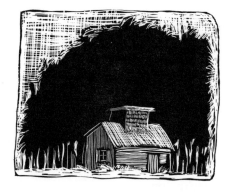

ZOO-ZOOS YOU'LL NEVER FORGET

First there was the dessert. Then came the treat. Next was the snack, and in the past decade, the munchie. Finally modern sweet-toothed inspiration has come up with something to top them all . . . the zoo-zoo. Frankly, I don't know where the term originated, but I know what it means to me. Zoo-zoos are those once-in-a-while, "welcome home," "happy birthday," "I love you" treats. They are very special, and usually are shared with family, friends, or other special people.

Desserts have become a matter-of-fact way to end a meal in our culture. They're simply whipped up, defrosted, or unwrapped.

Treats have become so accessible and so well advertised that it's all too easy to substitute them for other forms of personal "treatment." A foot rub, hot bath, or kind thought could be just as effective as that food reward.

Snacks are part of a fast-paced world. They are eaten when there is no time to eat. In fact snacks sometimes replace meals.

Munchies, the most recent of these sweet-toothed concepts, are things you munch on—unconsciously. Your mind might be somewhere else entirely, but when the munchies are brought out you might find yourself reaching for them and reaching for them, and reaching for them.

Zoo-zoos, whether they are simple or fancy are an occasion in themselves—worth waiting for, and only needed in small amounts. Here are some of our best, most favorite zoo-zoos.

AVOCADO MERINGUE PIE

Crust

¼ cup butter
1½ cups whole-wheat flour
dash of salt
ice water to mix

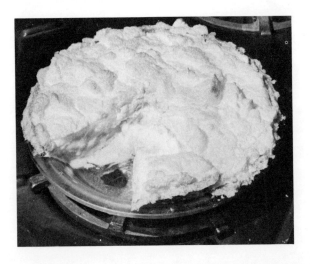

Mash butter into flour/salt mixture until flour becomes the size of large peas. Add enough ice water to moisten the flour and gather it into a ball (don't handle it too much—this causes a tough crust).

Roll dough out onto a floured board, making it large enough for an 8-inch pan. Bake at 350° for about 10 minutes or until brown.

Filling

1 large avocado
1 can (14 ounces) condensed goat's milk (or equivalent)
grated rind of 1 lime
½ cup fresh lime juice
2 egg yolks
dash of salt

Mash avocado well. Combine milk, lime rind, lime juice, beaten egg yolks, and salt. Stir until thickened. Fold in avocado. Put in pie shell and chill.

Cover with fresh lemon juice.

For meringue, add salt to 2 egg whites and whip till stiff.

Cover the pie with the meringue and put under the broiler for 2–3 minutes or until brown.

UNCOOKED TOFU CHEESECAKE

Ahead of time:

Press 2 cubes of fresh tofu for ½ hour. (To press tofu, wrap it in a dish towel, put it in a colander, and weight it down with a 5-pound honey tin, a jar full of water, or something else that will apply enough pressure to squeeze out water from the tofu. When the pressing is done, wring and squeeze the tofu in the dish towel to remove even more water.)

While tofu is being pressed, mix the crust. There's no need to cook it.

1½ cups granola
½ stick butter
1 cup toasted slivered almonds
¾ cup toasted shredded coconut

Mix and press into a 9-inch pan.

For the filling, combine the pressed and squeezed tofu with:

1 tablespoon carob powder
1 teaspoon vanilla
¼ teaspoon cinnamon
¾–1 cup honey
1 tablespoon tahini or sesame butter

Mix all ingredients until fluffy, then spoon into the crust, decorate, chill, and serve.

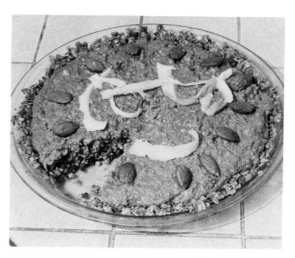

ALMOND JOY BARS

Combine and set aside:

½ cup fresh wheat flour
1 cup coarsely ground almonds
2 cups shredded coconut
pinch of salt

Cream:

¼ cup butter (½ stick)
1 cap Mexican vanilla (or 1 teaspoon regular
  vanilla)
½–¾ cup honey

Preheat oven to 325°. Mix dry ingredients into
butter/honey mix a little at a time. When it gets
too dry to stir add ¼ cup milk. Mix it up—pat
down with hands onto a cookie tray. Bake for
15–20 minutes.

Now, while it's in the oven, melt about 1 cup
honey and 1 cup carob powder together. When
bars come out of the oven top with the carob
sauce and sprinkle the tops with sliced almonds
cut into shapes, and ENJOY!!

(EDITOR'S NOTE: *You can use lemon or orange
juice to replace the milk, or try a nut milk for a
good healthy change! Make the dough into lots
of different and fancy shapes and top with whole
almonds. Delicious!!*)

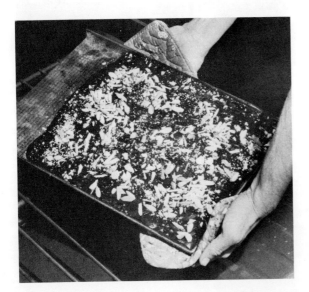

A Sweet Tooth Story

Once I lived on a farm, thirty miles from the
nearest town. After a full summer of blackberry
pies, apple pies, homemade ice cream, honey and
corn bread, honey and tea, honey and everything,
our sixty-pound honey tin was empty. We decided that rather than get more (the price had
just gone up) we'd do without it for a while.
There were plenty of sweet vegetables and fruits,
and we rediscovered the sweetness of grains. Before we knew it, we realized that we didn't miss
honey at all. Of course each trip to town offered
us all the indulgible treats, and I must admit that
the same farm now has six beehives, but the point
is, that by going without it for a while, we broke
the "honey habit." Now I enjoy occasional
sweets. The honey supply diminishes very slowly
and I feel much healthier—physically and emotionally. My sweet tooth has grown dormant from
lack of attention.   D.C.

CAPRICIOUS CARROT CAKE

by Joshua the Honey Bear

2 cups whole-wheat flour
2 teaspoons baking powder
¼ teaspoon vegetable salt
1 teaspoon cinnamon
3 eggs, separated
1 cup honey
½ cup vegetable oil
1 teaspoon vanilla
1½ cups grated raw carrots or carrot pulp
  from juicer
1 handful chopped walnuts
1 handful raisins

Preheat oven to 350°. Mix together flour, baking powder, salt, and cinnamon. In another bowl combine egg yolks, honey, oil, and vanilla. Add this slowly to dry ingredients. Add carrots, walnuts, and raisins, and finally fold in stiffly beaten egg whites. Bake in an oiled pan for 1¼ hours. It can be stored for weeks like a fruit cake if kept well wrapped and in a cool place.

CHRISTMAS DELIGHTS

CHRISTMAS COOKIES

¾ cup butter (or oil and butter)
1 cup honey
2 teaspoons baking powder
4 cups flour
2 teaspoons vanilla

Cream butter and honey, add rest of ingredients. Mix (knead a little), chill 1 hour. Roll on a floured board to about ⅛-inch thickness (can use a tall wine bottle if you don't have a rolling pin . . . works fine!). Cut out the cookies in your favorite design. Bake on an oiled sheet at 400° for 8–10 minutes till just getting brown.

RICE PUDDING

1 cup water
2 tablespoons agar-agar
2 tablespoons flax seeds
2 cups cooked rice
¼–½ cup honey
juice of ¼ lemon
1 teaspoon vanilla
nutmeg
cinnamon
ginger

Simmer water, agar-agar, and flax seeds 5 minutes. Mix with rest of ingredients. Refrigerate an hour or so before serving.

SUMMERTIME TREATS YOU CAN MAKE

by Suza Norton, with additions by the Well-Being *staff*

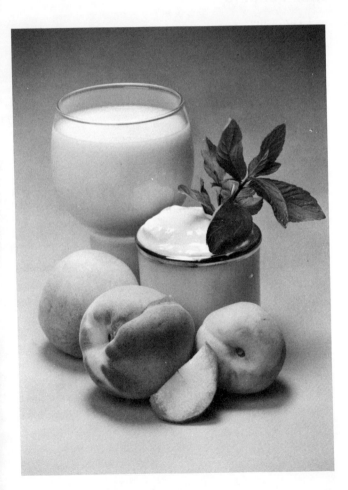

When your kids reach the age of Coke-consciousness (Pepsi de-generation)—that is, when they know how to put a quarter in the vending machine and out it comes—it's time to dream up some cold refreshing substitutes, preferably ones they can make themselves.

YOGHURT PINEAPPLE SHERBET: 1 cup crushed pineapple, 1 cup yoghurt. Put yoghurt in freezing tray and freeze slowly to a soft mush. Remove and stir in crushed pineapple and juice. Return to freezing compartment and freeze to soft consistency again. Stir or beat well and again freeze until solid, or eat as it is if you can't wait.

For variety use honey-sweetened mashed strawberries, raspberries, boysenberries, finely diced peaches, or very ripe apricots.

FROSTED BANANAS are an example of a popsicle-type alternative: use well-speckled ripe —but not mushy—bananas. Break in halves or thirds. Prepare a dip made of carob powder and water. Add water gradually to the carob powder to get a smooth consistency, not too fudgy or too thin. Roll the bananas right after peeling into this carob dip, coating well all over. (Can use tongs.) Then roll in finely grated coconut; insert popsicle sticks; place on cookie sheet or flat plate, and freeze. When frozen firm, package individually in airtight bags and store in the freezer so they're ready to go when the Good Humor truck dingles by.

And of course there are umpteen ways to make cool *summer fruit smoothies.* Teach your older youngsters which button does what on the blender and they'll quickly become smoothie experts.

Here are a few of our kid-kitchen-tested combinations:

Raw milk, frozen bananas (makes the smoothie very thick and rich), ripe apricots or other juicy fruit.

Finely shredded coconut, unsweetened canned or fresh pineapple chunks, milk or yoghurt.

Fresh orange juice and frozen bananas.

Juggle ingredients to suit your taste—experiment with different ways to make them thick and creamy. (Yoghurt, a little honey, and any juicy ripe fruit.)

If you don't have any frozen fruit on hand and the kids insist on an ice-cold smoothie, just add a few ice cubes.

An example of how to juggle the ingredients:

STRAWBERRY SMOOTHIE

2 cups fresh strawberries
2 tablespoons or less raw honey
2 cups milk
frozen bananas (or use frozen strawberries)

DATE/COCONUT SMOOTHIE: Put a few dates (according to desired sweetness) and a generous amount (experiment) of finely shredded unsweetened coconut in blender. Add just enough milk to cover blade. Blend until dates are completely "blended" (chopped until they disappear into the milk), add more milk—very frothy and delicious. Juggle the above amounts to suit your sweet tooth.

We have to add that we're not recommending any ice-cold concoctions as being ideal drinks. In general it's best to eat foods neither too hot nor too cold. But these smoothies are especially pleasing substitutes for the usual artificial sugary drinks sold at the local frosties.

You can make *natural soda pop* by combining natural, unsweetened fruit-juice concentrates with carbonated water. Mix to taste—about half and half is good. Both of these products are usually available at natural food stores. To make your own *ginger ale,* use:

3–4 ounces bruised fresh ginger root
4–5 cups honey
6 lemons, cut up, rind and all, minus the seeds

Place these ingredients in a large earthenware crock, or the jug from a water cooler. (This is handy to use as it has a spout for bottling later.) To this add:

4 gallons boiling water
2 tablespoons baking yeast which has been dissolved in about ¼ cup water

Cover the jug with cheesecloth so it can "breathe" while its natural carbonation develops. Let it stand for about 24 hours, then bottle. (You may want to strain it as you bottle.) I found that old wine bottles, washed and sterilized, with new corks, worked fine. Cork securely, but not too tightly, as it's better to blow your cork than to burst your bottle. Store bottles in a cold place: refrigerator, spring box, cellar, etc. The ale will ferment if left in a warmer environment, which isn't a bad idea. But if you're making it for your kids . . .

MINTY PEACH CLOUD

1 cup yoghurt
1 sliced peach
1 sprig mint
1 tablespoon of honey or more

Chop, glop, whiz, and bliss out.

QUICK GINGER ALE

6 teaspoons honey
1 quart Calistoga mineral water
2 teaspoons fresh ginger, grated extremely fine
   (or ½ cup ginger tea)
⅛ teaspoon cayenne
1 lemon or 2 small limes

First stir honey in a little heated spring water;
then mix all together.

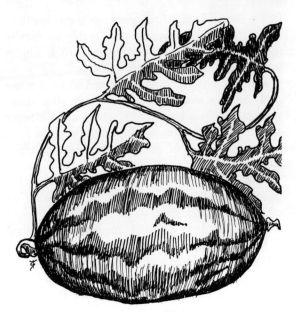

SOFT DRINKS:
Were They Always This Bad?

by Marianne Seidel

Since the birth of Coca-Cola in 1886, soft drinks undoubtedly have become one of the most widely consumed commercial products. Billions of dollars have been spent luring "those who think young" to enjoy "the pause that refreshes." In spite of advertising persistence, many of the "Now generation" are questioning the validity of these slogans and are researching the effects of the additives in soft drinks.

Georgia pharmacist "Doc" Pemberton's original Coca-Cola syrup was a boiled mixture of extracts from kola nuts and untreated coca leaf with fruit syrup. He first sold his syrup to Jacob's Drug Store in Atlanta. It was here that Coca-Cola was given its name and the fountain man's accidental addition of soda water changed the flat drink to a zesty pick-me-up. Twenty-five gallons of syrup were sold the first year for fifty dollars.

The combination of coca leaf's anesthetic effect on the stomach, reducing hunger pangs, and kola nut's reputation as a water purifier, strengthener, hangover cure, and "love potion," was thought to be an ideal tonic. In the 1890s Coca-Cola was promoted as a nerve and brain tonic: "Relieves mental or physical exhaustion," and "offers relief from biliousness (sluggish liver), indigestion, mention exhaustion, and nervous headache."* Sales jumped to $144,000—48,427 gallons of syrup in 1893. In 1968, Coca-Cola sales were six billion gallons—one trillion drinks—and the company boasted that at least 95,000,000 drinks were consumed each day.

America's concern about the long-term use of patent medicines and opiates resulted in the 1906 Food and Drug Act. Coca-Cola foresaw such legislation and removed the minute amounts of cocaine (known for its stimulating effects on the nervous system) from each coca leaf.

By 1916, when a thousand bottlers were serving Coca-Cola to all the U.S. states, other soft drinks, such as Hires Root Beer, 7-Up, Dr. Pepper, Orange Crush, Royal Crown Cola, Pepsi-Cola, and Nehi were manufactured from a variety of natural syrups and soda water. Others, like Coo-Coo, Kold Kup, Bruce's Juices, and Tip 2 Lip, never caught on.

* Lawrence Dietz, *Soda Pop* (New York: Simon and Schuster, 1973), p. 18.

THEN CAME THE ADDITIVES

Soft drink labels now, however, display a variety of multisyllabled chemical additives which have a variety of functions, and natural and synthetic flavorings and colorings, but not all ingredients must be listed. Books are now in print for consumer use explaining the functions of additives. These can be found in the library or health and natural food stores (see Bibliography).

There are at least twenty-five natural and synthetic soft drink flavorings, including caffeine (also used as a preservative), which is obtained as a by-product from caffeine-free coffee. Colorings or dyes are used such as brown caramel (burnt sugar) and coal-tar derivatives such as sodium chloride. A non-nutritive sweetener such as saccharin (300 times sweeter than sugar), which is used in diet drinks, leaves a bitter aftertaste. These sweeteners leave the drink without body, which must be replaced with a water retainer like sodium-alginate, or cellulose gums, or pectins. Of course sugar is widely used as a sweetener. The remainder of the many additives consist mainly of:

anti-foaming agents like polysorbate 80 or dimethyl polysiloxane;
color fixatives like patchouly oil;
sequestrants, which prevent clouding and are also preservatives, like calcium disodium;
buffers or acidulants, which control the acidity, like phosphoric acid;
preservatives and anti-oxidants and brominated vegetable oils, which adjust the density of essential oils, keeping the drink clear.

Many of the additives widely used can be found on the FDA's priority list to study for mutagenic (causing biologic mutation), teratogenic (fetal deforming), subacute (disease causing), and reproductive effects. Many chemical additives are feared to be carcinogenic (cancer causing). (See Winter's *Consumer's Dictionary.*) Studies are finding that hyperactivity in children is often traced to chemical additives, as are other problems such as birth defects, diabetes, brain damage, intestinal disorders, hypothalamus, liver, heart, and kidney disease.

Alternatives are offered by a few food manufacturers who are concerned with quality and are returning to old-fashioned simplicity and taste. Look in the health or natural food store refrigerator for Health Maid Root Beer, Apple Rush, Hopping's Honey Soda, Osceola's Creme Cola or Spruce Root Beer, or root beer made by L & A Juice Company (partial list).

BIBLIOGRAPHY AND REFERENCE

Benarde, Dr. Melvin A. *The Chemicals We Eat.* New York: American Heritage Press, 1971.

Dietz, Lawrence. *Soda Pop.* New York: Simon and Schuster, 1973.

Verrett, Jacqueline, and Carper, Jean. *Eating May Be Hazardous to Your Health.* New York: Simon and Schuster, 1974; Anchor Press/Doubleday, 1975.

Winter, Ruth. *A Consumer's Dictionary of Food Additives.* New York: Crown Publishers, Inc., 1972.

NOURISHING NURSING MOTHERS

by Karen Shultz

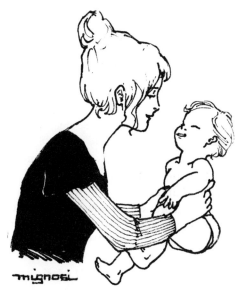

Most aware young mothers are lovingly conscientious about the quality of their prenatal diet. The ever-increasing size of the abdomen is an obvious reminder that good food is essential for the growing fetus. However, many of these same women—later overwhelmed by the actual birth and subsequent care of the child—"forget" that an *even higher quality diet* is required by the lactating mother. No other member of the human race has such acute nutritional demands!

More often than not, the baby has had its fill of breast milk early in the morning before mother has had a chance to eat *anything*. And fatigue and irritability can arise during the day without a superior breast-feeding regimen. If too few calories are consumed by the mother, her dietary and body protein will be used for caloric needs. Calcium and phosphorus can be leeched from her bones if her diet just isn't making it. (The situation is more crucial if a woman has birthed and nursed other children, because she may have developed a depletion of minerals—or negative calcium balance—due to repeated past demands upon her body. The breast-feeding experience is so beautiful it should not be disturbed by an inadequate diet. And this doesn't mean that a lot of money need be laid out for special foods, but that a few rules of thumb be followed.

It is important to remember that breast-milk production appropriates an *extra* 1,000–1,500 calories per day. This brings the total requirement to 3,000 calories each day to maintain the nursing mother and her milk supply. Without careful planning, the need for extra calories may create random selection of non-nourishing foods. Eating sugars, starches, and fatty foods does little but increase the saturated-fat content of the breast milk. While totally breast-feeding my infant, I am ravenously hungry! So I grab a few handfuls of almonds and raisins when I'm on the run. Nuts, sunflower seeds, cheese, and fruits are convenient milk-building snacks which help give the additional protein and vitamins that are needed.

MORE PROTEIN

The requirements for protein, vitamins, and minerals go way up as does the need for extra calories. It is a good idea to get about ninety grams of protein every day. This isn't always easy in a vegetarian family, and it takes a little foresight. I've been making a habit of eating ½ cup of cottage cheese (twenty grams protein) and ¼ cup of brewer's yeast (twenty grams protein) before I leave for errands in the morning. Then I know that I am well on my way to gaining my total of ninety grams of protein, the balance of which I'll pick up later in the day. Main meals can revolve around high-protein soybeans and soy derivatives such as tofu, soy flour, and soy milk.

Speaking of nutritional yeast, it is *the* food for the nursing mother. She needs a balanced source of B vitamins for her milk and her energy reserve, and yeast is the best provider, hands down! Mothers I know report less fatigue and a better milk flow by using brewer's yeast each day. One fourth cup, or four tablespoons, is a reasonable amount. Try yeast in pineapple juice if you just can't take it straight.

MORE CALCIUM

At no other time in life does a person need more calcium. Many breast-feeding women have a negative calcium balance. Calcium can be most easily provided by drinking one quart of raw milk daily, with the addition of one teaspoon calcium lactate; plus Formula ⚹82. It is a misconception, however, that dairy products are the only reliable source. Sesame tahini is an excellent calcium food that should be used everyday (with hulls). And the mother's high-calcium requirement can be met, in part, by eating steamed garden greens. These are highest in calcium in the following order: lamb's quarters, turnip, dandelion, mustard, and collard greens. Dried sea vegetables are another mineral-rich food that can be added to the nursing regimen. Yeast 500—which is fortified with calcium—comes to the rescue again! Five tablespoons will supply all the calcium food that should be used every day.

These basic foods must be fortified with generous amounts of fresh fruits and vegetables. Aim for six servings of fruits and vegetables every day —alfalfa sprouts are especially beneficial. Note that onions, garlic, cabbage, cauliflower, broccoli, and Brussels sprouts *may* cause gas in *some* babies.

And there is a particularly enjoyable method of adding a little Vitamin D to breast milk— frequent sunbathing! It's good for the breasts too. For good measure, I have added a complete vegetarian vitamin to my breast-feeding regimen, at a cost of about six cents per day.

FOR MORE MILK

My nursing friends and I are constantly thirsty! The liquid intake naturally increases with breast-feeding. Drinking three quarts of various liquids throughout the day should be quite adequate. An ideal distribution of liquids would be:

1 quart raw milk
1 quart fruit or vegetable juices
1 quart pure water or herbal teas

Some herbs that are "galactagogues"—that is, capable of promoting the flow of milk—are fennel seed, borage seed and leaves, and blessed thistle. A mother might want to drink something a few minutes before breast-feeding, or perhaps during nursing itself. If the urine becomes dark and concentrated, *more* liquids are needed.

Most important of all, don't forget that a healthy, relaxed outlook on life, accompanied by enough rest, will make the nursing experience that much more pleasant for you and your child. Your love comes right through your milk along with all the other good things.

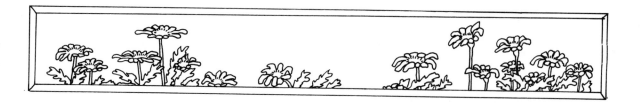

HERBAL COFFEE BREAKS:
They're Catching On!

by Allan Jaklich

Coffee is a heavy-duty herb . . . stimulating, addicting, and powerfully laxative. Many Americans use it habitually, consuming on the average of seventeen pounds per person each year. Some folks would never even consider that coffee might be contributing to some of their health problems. Even if you never use coffee/caffeine, you may find an occasional hot, steaming brew made from a robust blend of fine herbs and spices a pleasing break . . . maybe even healthful. For those who want to explore alternatives to coffee, there are many delicious and/or stimulating herbal beverages to choose from. Maybe if we all start appreciating the herbs that grow right outside our doors, the South Americans will start planting soybeans instead of coffee trees.

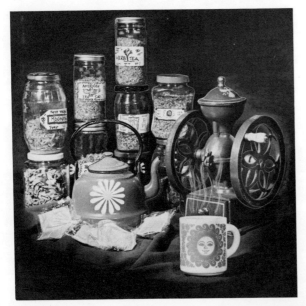

When I left the city behind to live at a mountain herb farm three years ago, I left coffee behind as well. It was then that I began to experience the subtle qualities of the many other herbal teas: burdock, chamomile, comfrey, the mints, mugwort, yerba santa, etc. Now that I'm back in the city's high-speed energy, coffee is only one of the many herbal beverages I choose from for my "herb breaks."

Coffee and other caffeine drinks are strong medicine. Fifty years ago William Boericke, both a doctor of medicine and professor of homeopathy, wrote that caffeine "raises the blood pressure, increases the pulse rate, and stimulates the heart muscles; hence a support in extreme feebleness or threatened failure." That's why caffeine is used as an antidote to snake bite and narcotic poisoning

. . . it's such a powerful stimulant that it staves off coma!

In general, caffeine is considered detrimental for folks with a weak liver, low blood sugar (hypoglycemia), or glaucoma . . . and adding milk and/or honey only worsens the effect.

What caffeine does is stimulate the endocrine glands, mostly the adrenals which release blood sugar, giving us a temporary lift. But what's more, caffeine is member of the same alkaloid chemical group as morphine, nicotine, cocaine, and strychnine—all having addictive properties. So with daily use we develop a tolerance to the stimulation. Our glands lose their ability to act naturally. So we *need* the stimulation.

That means that after habitual use, coming off coffee and other caffeine beverages will produce withdrawal symptoms as built-up toxins are released from the body. As Dr. Henry Bieler says in his book *Food Is Your Best Medicine,* "You feel fatigued, headache-y, depressed, so you drink more coffee to get through the day."

Coffee/caffeine can be psychologically as well as physically addictive. A regular dose of caffeine can make it easier to ignore bothersome feelings— physical *and* emotional. The two seem, after all, to go hand in hand. Keeping ourselves continually stimulated may mask symptoms, but only delays dealing with the causes.

When I overdo the caffeine—whether from coffee or other herbs—I awake with a fuzzy head and poor digestion. To remedy this I start the morning with one of the following herbs: ginseng, gotu kola, goldenseal, cayenne. (These, along with regular fasting, vigorous exercise, dry skin brushing, ending baths and showers with a cold blast, and generally improving the diet should help any "coffee-holic" recover while kicking the caffeine habit.)

Coffee also contains tannic acid, an effective laxative. And just as our glands learn to tolerate and need constant stimulation, with habitual use of coffee/tannic acid our bowels learn to tolerate and need its laxative effect. No wonder so many folks need a cup of coffee to start the day right!

Arguments, of course, rage on all sides of the coffee/caffeine issue. Dr. Bernard Jensen goes so far as to say coffee has no place in the diet, while Carlton Fredericks, author of *Low Blood Sugar and You,* says, "If coffee does not overstimulate you, and if you do not have hypoglycemia or a tendency toward it, this favorite beverage can hold its place in your nutritional scheme of things."

The answer for each of us—"coffee-holics" and "tea-totalers" included—is to know how much, if any, we can handle and still maintain our health.

In my case, if I drink coffee several days in a row I begin to need a cup of it to wake up each day. But I also get jittery, irritable, and develop sore insides . . . so I'm forced to lay off the coffee. As a result, I use coffee and other caffeine beverages only occasionally—when I need to stay up late, or need a quick laxative.

In between my occasional cups of coffee (I drink it maybe once a week) I enjoy plenty of other hot herb drinks, for various effects.

STIMULANTS

Black tea (fermented green tea leaves) contains about the same amount of caffeine and tannic acid as coffee. The taste is a refreshing change, and it definitely gives a lift. Some friends drink it regularly, with milk and honey. But like coffee, it is strong medicine for me, so I have it only occasionally.

Caffeine and Birth

The Center for Science in the Public Interest has demanded that the Department of Health, Education, and Welfare advise women in the first few months of pregnancy to cut down on coffee, tea, and nonprescription drugs that contain the stimulant caffeine. "It is clear," the center said in a letter to HEW, "that caffeine causes birth defects when animals are exposed to moderately high levels of the drug," and "the levels that caused defects in three (animal) studies are levels to which a small minority of pregnant women is likely to be exposed." Meanwhile, the center has also demanded that HEW closely study the relationship between caffeine and human birth defects, miscarriage, and infertility, and also alert physicians. Information from *Ms.* Magazine

Yerba maté, from South America, is claimed to be beneficial for headache, migraine, neuralgia, and insomnia! . . . even though it too contains caffeine (it is less stimulating and astringent than coffee, however). It even adds vitamin C to the diet. A mildly stimulating and mild-tasting tea.

Celestial Seasonings has blended black tea and yerba maté into "Morning Thunder." They recommend not boiling it, and even say steeping longer than four minutes increases the tannic acid. Seems true for coffee too.

Guarana and kola nuts are herbs I've yet to experience. Guarana has three times more caffeine than coffee! A friend says it can be useful in special situations, like all-night driving, but too much caffeine will cause negative effects (plus it tastes awful). Kola nuts (100 tons are imported from West Africa each year to go into our cola drinks) by weight contain more caffeine than coffee berries. A friend has ground them up to make—with mint—a tasty, stimulating tea.

LAXATIVES

If I need a laxative but want to avoid caffeine, I make a cup of strong licorice root tea (also great for coughs and sore throats). Goldenseal usually puts my gastrointestinal tract through the necessary changes as well. A friend recommends buckthorn bark highly. No laxative should be used habitually, of course.

Herbal "Pick Me Ups"

Caffeine Herbs
Guarana (*Paullinia cupana*)
Kola nuts (*kola vera*)
Coffee (*Coffea arabica*)
Tea (*Thea sinesis*)
Yerba maté (*Ilex paraguayensis*)

Other Stimulants
Ginseng (*Panax quinquefolium*)
Cayenne (*Capsicum frutescens*)
Ginger (*Zingiber officinale*)
Gotu kola (*Hydrocotyle asiatica*)

Rich and Dark Blends
"Naturally Good" "Postum"
"Roastaroma Mocha Spice" "Pero"

Laxatives
Licorice (*Glycyrrhiza glabra*)
Goldenseal (*Hydrastis canadensis*)
Buckthorn bark (*Cascara sagrada*)

Do-it-yourself Blends
Burdock, dandelion and chicory roots, carob, barley, soybeans, carrots, and/or figs. Roast in a slow oven until dark brown, turning often. Then grind.

Take an Herb to Lunch . . . Really!

Go to most any restaurant and you will be faced with the following selection of hot beverages: coffee, Lipton's (or a similar brand) or Constant Comment Tea, and chocolate . . . all stimulants (cocoa and chocolate contain theobromine, similar to caffeine in effect).

Ask for "herb tea" at the typical restaurant and it's likely the waitress will act as though you have spoken in a foreign tongue. But persevere! With the price of coffee continually rising, and the popularity of other kinds of hot herbal beverages increasing, it seems only a matter of time until cafe owners will recognize an opportunity waiting to be met.

Meanwhile, here's what you can do to get a healthy, hot drink when eating out.

1. If they don't have your favorite herb tea, ask for a pot of hot water anyway. I've seen waitresses surprised and interested, but rarely upset at serving just hot water. Chances are you won't even be charged.

2. If you forget to bring your own tea bags, ask for some fresh lemon (maybe even honey) and make your own healthful hot drink alternative (suggestions compliments of Dean).

3. If you get into the habit of carrying your own box of herb tea bags when you travel (I carry a jar of ginseng extract) you'll always have a good cup of tea, plus have the chance to show restaurant owners what lots of folks are drinking for a hot beverage these days. They'll get the message!

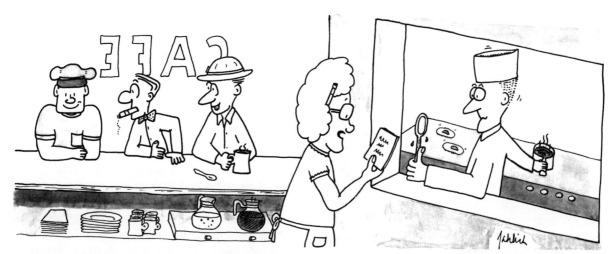

"He's asking for someone called 'Herb' Tea."

STIMULATION WITHOUT CAFFEINE

There also are herbs that stimulate/tone in a different way.

Ginseng is one of my favorites. Much has been written about this rejuvenating root (did you know that most of the ginseng grown in the United States is exported to Asia, where it is a major herb?). To me it is only slightly stimulating, and seems more of a tonic . . . refreshing, with no side effects that I've noticed. Of course it's expensive but coffee is no bargain either.

Cayenne surprisingly tones rather than burns my insides, leaving me internally "stimulated." Besides using it on my food, I occasionally start the day taking a half teaspoon mixed in a half glass of pure water. Others add it to teas, and believe it or not it's good! You may be more sensitive so if you want to try cayenne for the first time, start with small amounts until you find your right dosage.

Ginger, another fine "spice" in foods, also makes an excellent, circulation-stimulating tea. Sliced thin and simmered (the longer the stronger) it is especially delicious with a little milk and honey. Its effect is also subtle, but sipped as the first beverage in the morning it certainly gives a lift. Like cayenne, ginger benefits both circulation and digestion.

Yogi tea is one of the blends we drink on herbal coffee breaks at the *Well-Being* office; it smells so good when it's brewing. It can be blended a number of ways, using cinnamon, clove, ginger, allspice, cardamom, licorice, star anise, etc. Percentages of ingredients and brewing time will make big differences, so experiment.

Mu tea is another favorite, usually prepackaged, easy to prepare, and rebrewable without becoming too strong. There are a number of mu blends on the market, usually made with oriental herbs.

(One great advantage to using herb seeds, roots, and barks—anise, burdock, sassafras—for teas is that they can be brewed twice or more, adding pure water as needed. You can always keep a pot of hot tea brewin' at the office/party.)

DARK AND RICH BLENDS

When I want a good, hot coffee substitute— something more substantial than say, peppermint but without stimulation—I drink one of my two current favorites.

Naturally good—raw and roasted chicory root, roasted dandelion root, sarsaparilla, burdock root, and licorice root. This blend from Magic Forest Earth Arts has, like ginseng, a decidedly medicinal or tonic flavor, almost thick. It is a tonic for the organs; I acquired a taste for it while taking it for my health. Now I like it!

Roastaroma mocha spice—barley, malt, chicory root, carob, and dandelion root . . . all roasted, plus cinnamon, allspice, ginger, and Chinese star anise. Another Celestial Seasonings tea, and great with milk and honey.

Pero, Postum, and decaffeinated coffee—I've tried them. Pero and Postum are powdered, made mostly from grains. They are convenient . . . just add hot water. Decaf coffee tastes O.K., but since I heard it's made by soaking coffee beans in a "solvent," then distilling with steam, I have decided not to drink it. I like my foods unadulterated.

DO-IT-YOURSELF BLENDS

Of course you can blend your own coffee substitutes too (and if you discover a particularly pleasing and/or healthful beverage for your herbal breaks, please share it with us). In addition to the herbs and grains mentioned earlier you might try roasted soybeans, carrots, English oak acorns, or figs.

Coffee in moderation has its place among herbs. I wrote the first draft of this story one evening after grinding, brewing, and drinking two cups of Guatemalan (just for the first-hand experience). When I finished after midnight I was still buzzin'. Next day my insides said I'd had enough. That's O.K. There are plenty of delicious herb beverages to enjoy.

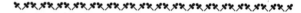

Nickel Coffee

Philippe's Original Sandwich Shop in downtown L.A. still serves coffee for a nickel a cup . . . just because that's the way Grandpa wanted it. Co-owner Bill Binder says, "The actual coffee costs us about 3.8 cents a cup. But then you have to figure in the labor, plus the dishwater used, the cream and sugar (honey, that is.—eds.), the breakage, things like that." He adds, "Well, it makes you shake your head when you figure what the other restaurants are getting away with."

(Perhaps the other restaurants use a more expensive blend of dishwater.)

New West magazine

HERB TEAS THAT SUPPLY ESSENTIAL NUTRIENTS

by William LeSassier

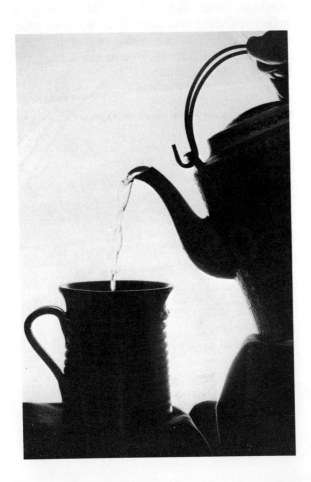

The most highly valued herbs for the building cycle in the body are called nutritive herbs. Your richest forms of nutrition are for the most part found either in plants that are aquatic or trees. These plants have access to trace elements preserved in either stones or deep earth. The nutritive herbs are extremely low in toxicity, in fact so low that there are almost no counterindications for their use. A person would have to take a ridiculous amount of these herbs for them to have a toxic effect. Some of these herbs affect a particular system, but their effect is still almost totally nutritive.

Slippery elm contains trace elements for the brain. Trees contain the deepest roots and can bring much into the surface of the earth. Slippery elm has some of the highest nutrition counts of any food. It helps stabilize the emotions and has rejuvenating effect on the glandular system. It is fattening, good for debilitated systems. 1 tablespoon daily.

Alfalfa has literally hundreds of values, incredibly rich in magnesium and most minerals. It has very deep root structures. It inhibits clotting, prevents senility; however, it does thin the blood so would not be good excessively in winter as it could contribute to cold hands and feet. Alfalfa contains cyanocobalamin, the vitamin B$_{12}$. 1 tablespoon daily.

Oat straw rich in silicon, good for bladder and kidneys. Helps in calcium imbalances. 2 tablespoons daily.

Irish moss contains iodine, many trace elements, excellent for lungs and antibiotic function. 2 tablespoons daily.

Yellow dock root contains natural iron and balanced copper. It is beneficial to colon and blood. 1 tablespoon daily.

Watercress excellent for the blood. Contains iron, sodium, copper, and trace elements found in highly mineralized waters of different locations. 2 tablespoons daily.

Nettle high in iron, magnesium, potassium. Also picks up highly mineralized waters. Contains tremendous life energy. Excellent for weak people. Helps for clotting and has a stabilizing effect on the kidneys. Helps against anemia, excessive menstruation, etc. Will reduce weight, but do not use if terribly underweight. 1 tablespoon daily.

Chickweed high in calcium. Excellent for lungs and debilitation—good for excessive sweating. Nutritive dried or fresh.

Raspberry leaves extremely high in calcium/ magnesium balance. Strengthens joints and tendons. Good for kidneys (to stabilize excessive flow). Used in birth tonics. I call it vegetable dolomite. 1 teaspoon daily.

Lemon grass rich in silica, for bladder and kidneys. Cools the system, used in the summer.

Hibiscus rich in vitamin C—also cools the system and is good in the summer. Not used in the winter as it is too cooling.

Rose hips rich in vitamin C and bioflavonoids. Do not boil rose hips or hibiscus as it destroys the vitamin C.

Here are some teas for various deficiencies. They are not designed to replace supplements but rather to enhance absorption of minerals from dietary and other natural sources. Plants contain minerals that are readily absorbed and therefore readily used.

CALCIUM TEA

1 part chamomile
1 part borage
½ part comfrey
1 part oat straw

Combine by size. These can either be powdered and ground on food (1 tablespoon daily) or can be steeped 1 tablespoon per cup for 30–45 minutes. The tea is good for menstrual cramps, nursing mothers, heart patients, etc.

TRACE ELEMENT TEA

⅓ part slippery elm
1 part bladder wrack
1 part watercress
1 part alfalfa
1 part nettle
1 part fennel

Mix and sweeten with maple sugar (organically grown).

POTASSIUM TEA

(Don't take salt or sodium if you have potassium deficiency.)

1 part plantain (dried leaves)
1 part chickweed leaves
1 part blackberry leaves
1 part carrot leaves
1 part fennel leaves

Combine 1 tablespoon daily as a tea or powder on food.

IRON TEA

1 part yellow dock
1 part nettle
1 part dried beet powder
1 part dried watercress
1 part parsley
1 part dandelion root
1 part dulse

Combine by size 1 tablespoon daily as a tea or powder or food.

Other wild-food substances that have trace elements in them: lamb's quarters, elderberries, Oregon grape berries, edible chrysanthemums, chimaja, wild carrot, spearmint, wild lettuce, acorns, fresh elder flowers, wild berries, fiddlehead ferns (western and eastern bracken), purslane (high in oxalic acid), lomatum root, fresh clover blossoms, vidler leaves, chickweed, wild onions, malva.

Wild foods contain much vitality and should be eaten whenever possible.

MEDICINAL USES FOR CULINARY HERBS

compiled by Ginny Clark

Allspice aromatic, carminative, stimulant. Added to a bath, allspice is said to have anesthetic effects.

Anise antispasmodic, aromatic, carminative, digestive, expectorant, stimulant, stomachic, tonic. Anise promotes digestion, improves appetite, alleviates cramps and nausea and relieves flatulence, especially in infants. Promotes the flow of milk in nursing mothers. Promotes menstruation. For insomina, steep a few seeds in warm milk before going to bed. It is said that a strong decoction applied to the head will kill lice.

Basil antispasmodic, carminative, stomachic. Used for stomach cramps, gastric catarrh, and excessive vomiting. Hindus use this holy herb to disinfect their homes. Used externally, it draws out poisons from insect bites. Has been used for antidote for hemp overdose.

Bay laurel astringent, carminative, digestive, stomachic. Stimulating to digestion. Poultice good for chest colds or insect stings.

Bean (dry pods before fully matured) diuretic, useful in dropsy, kidney and bladder trouble, uric acid accumulations, and loss of albumin in urine during pregnancy. Bean meal applied directly to cases of eczema, eruptions, and itching is beneficial.

Caraway antispasmodic, carminative, emmenagogue, expectorant. Use caraway for flatulent colic, particularly in infants and also to relieve nausea. Promotes menstruation, relieves uterine cramps, promotes milk in mothers, and is mildly expectorant. Powdered seed used as a poultice for bruises.

Cardamom carminative, stimulant, stomachic. Cardamom is rarely used alone but rather in combination with other herbs.

Cayenne stimulant, digestive, irritant, sialagogue, tonic. Stimulating both internally and externally. Care should be taken when taking cayenne in capsules as it can cause catarrh when taken in large doses. Produces heat for cold feet when put into socks.

Celery Plant: diuretic, emmenagogue. Seed: carminative, sedative. Celery promotes sleep. Should be taken in moderate amounts when pregnant as it will promote menstruation in larger doses. Very helpful in clearing skin problems. Good poultice for burns, etc. If crushed and applied to poison oak, celery will help take away the swelling.

Chervil digestive, diuretic, expectorant, stimulant.

Chives digestive—contain iron, thus may be helpful in anemia.

Cinnamon stomachic, carminative, mildly astringent, emmenagogue. Useful in diarrhea, nausea, vomiting, and flatulence. The tincture is useful in uterine hemorrhage.

Clove anodyne, antiemetic, antiseptic. Good for toothache and teething babies if dropped in cavity or rubbed on gums.

Coriander antispasmodic, aromatic, carminative, stomachic. Good addition to herbal preparations to improve taste. Will stop griping caused by laxatives and will expel gas. Young plants make good salad greens. The greens are called cilantro.

Cucumber aperient, diuretic. Important in heart and kidney problems because of its ability to eliminate water from the body. Also helps dissolve uric acid accumulations. Good for chronic constipation. Cucumber juice is beneficial for intestines, lungs, kidneys, skin. Good local application for burns. Cooling and soothing to skin.

Dill antispasmodic, calmative, carminative, diuretic, stomachic. Increases mother's milk especially when combined with anise, coriander, fennel, and caraway. Chew the seeds for bad breath. Will expel gas.

Fennel antispasmodic, aromatic, carminative, diuretic, expectorant, stimulant, stomachic. Increases mother's milk. Helps relieve abdominal cramps, flatulence, and will expel mucus. Will stop griping from laxatives. Similar in almost every respect to anise.

Fenugreek expectorant, mucilagenous, restorative. Good for people recovering from illness. Use as a gargle for sore throat. Excellent poultice for wounds.

Flax demulcent, emollient, purgative. A decoction of seeds is used for coughs, catarrh, lung and chest problems, digestive and urinary disorders. Excellent poultice for sores.

Garlic antiseptic, anthelmintic, antispasmodic, carminative, digestive, diuretic, expectorant, febrifuge. To break a fever in a small child or baby, oil the bottom of the child's feet, rub garlic juice (from pressed garlic) on the soles of the feet, taking care to wipe off any chunks of garlic pulp. Put socks on the child, bundle him up, put him to bed. The garlic will be absorbed into his system and he will sweat. Garlic stimulates peristaltic action in the bowels. The tincture is good for coughs, sore throat, diarrhea. Good for treating worms when given with a laxative. Use a slice of garlic to relieve painful gums temporarily.

Ginger adjuvant, carminative, diaphoretic, stimulant. Promotes cleansing of the system through perspiration. Good for suppressed menstruation, flatulent colic, and to stimulate flow of saliva.

Horseradish diuretic, rubifacient, stomachic. Use in colic, bladder infections, use externally to stimulate circulation. Good for sinus conditions and at the first sign of a cold. Grate ½ teaspoon, add a drop of lemon juice, and hold in the mouth. Inhale up through back of nose. Don't overdo it, though.

Lettuce anodyne, antispasmodic, expectorant, sedative. When lettuce has gone to seed it contains a milky substance which is sedative. Good for insomnia and nervous conditions. Useful in coughs, asthma, and cramps. Excellent green poultice for bruises and burns.

Marjoram antispasmodic, calmative, diaphoretic, expectorant, stomachic, tonic. Good for colic in children.

Nutmeg aromatic, carminative, stimulant. Small amount of the oil aids digestion and stops flatulence. Used in hot foot baths.

Oregano antispasmodic, calmative, carminative, diaphoretic, expectorant, stomachic, tonic, antiseptic. Good for headaches, nervousness, upset stomach and indigestion. Oil dropped in cavity is good for toothache. Calming bath additive. Leaves makes good sleep pillow for insomnia. Mexicans use it as an antiseptic for cuts and wounds.

Parsley antispasmodic, carminative, diuretic, emmenagogue, expectorant. Excellent for jaundice, fevers, stones in kidneys, difficult urination. Helps prevent illness. Good source of vitamins A and B. Seeds are a febrifuge.

Potato Excellent poultice when grated and applied fresh to old sores and ulcers. Poultice must be changed often and a new one applied. Also useful for burns and scalds. Hot potato water is good for swellings and painful areas. Never peel a potato as most nutrients are in the peel. Mealy flour made from baked potatoes is a good application for frostbite. Raw potato juice is good for gout, rheumatism.

Rosemary antispasmodic, emmenagogue, stimulant, stomachic. Old remedy for colds, colic, and nerves (good for headache). Good gargle for sore throat. Aids digestion. Good for female problems but should be avoided by pregnant women.

Sage antispasmodic, astringent, carminative. Cold tea is used to dry up mother's milk. Good in lung troubles. Inhale vapors to treat asthma. Cleansing for old sores and ulcers. Soothing to nerves. Excellent hair rinse for dandruff. Given hot will produce sweat. When signs of cold begin, drink sage tea (2 cups), get into hot bath, and sweat. Good for baby's colic and strengthening digestive tract.

Salt (crude sea salt, or earth salt). Use as a mouthwash for infections of the gums. Use hot salt pack for relief. A salt glow is good for low blood pressure and sluggishness. It is a vigorous rub with hot wet salt after a cold shower. Contains trace minerals.

Savory astringent, carminative, expectorant, stimulant. Good remedy for stomach disorders. Good in diarrhea. Will stop bleeding of wounds.

Tarragon diuretic, emmenagogue, stomachic.

Thyme anthelmintic, antispasmodic, carminative, expectorant, sedative, emmenagogue. Will cause perspiration when taken hot. Taken cold, good for diarrhea, cramps in the stomach, gas and lung troubles. Should be taken in moderate amounts when pregnant as it will promote menstruation in larger doses.

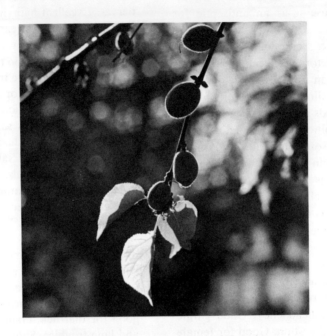

"Don't worry about your life and what
You are to eat, nor about your body
And how you are to clothe it. For
life means more than food, and the
body means more than clothing."

MATTHEW 6:25

III

WHAT IS NATURAL
HEALTH CARE?

WHAT IS NATURAL HEALTH CARE?

As we witness a growing interest in energy sources, food-growing techniques, and technologies which act in harmony with nature, we are also seeing a return to working with nature, and not against it, in health care. We are caretakers of our planet and of our bodies. Natural health care seeks to understand human ecology and cultivate, rather than deplete, the body's natural resources.

When we observe ourselves as part of nature, the operation manual for healthful living becomes clear. Nature offers us plants, water, sunshine, and the very earth—healing clays, for us to use in the care of our health. Humankind has developed numerous methods for using the body itself, through manipulations of joints, relaxation of muscles, or stimulation of points, to correct many imbalances which can and do occur in our everyday life.

Many of the techniques which fall into the category of natural health care have come to us from folk medicine. They are our heritage of common sense in caring for ourselves. Scientific inquiry can play a helpful hand in the development of quality natural health care for the masses, but only if the science of individual human ecology is studied deeply and seriously.

Health care has become far more complicated than it needs to be, with people ingesting materials that do not naturally exist in the same world as man, but were created by the human mind to correct what the human mind thought was happening. This complicated approach has had its successes. Some of us wouldn't be here today if "medicine" hadn't saved our lives. Yet despite the drama of man-made miracles and their benefits, we are left stranded and isolated in nature if we do not cultivate both a faith in and a knowledge of it. If you want to take pictures with a camera you don't put typing paper in it, you use what the creator of the camera intended, film. In a similar way plants, water, clay, and the like are what our Creator intended for us to put into our bodies in order to function at our best.

"Wholistic" or "holistic" are the terms which are nowadays being loosely applied to any technique, teacher, or organization which acknowledges and works with the dynamic interaction between the body, mind, and spirit. They can be just as misleading as the terms "natural" and "organic" have become on the labels of supermarket goods. Consumers of medical care need to become educated enough about their own body, mind, and spirit to look beyond the name and read the label. Medical education, on the other hand, is becoming broader and more diversified. If the consumers and providers of health care work together to develop fair and responsible medical laws we will have doctors of chiropractic, doctors of naturopathy, midwives, herbalists, medical doctors, homeopaths, and the like practicing their particular specialties within the limits of their own professions, but in a much less limited way than is now allowed. There is a great need today for "medical ecologists" and for choice in health care. As we are discovering a wide variety of ways to generate energy ecologically, so too are we discovering a wide variety of natural health-care methods. Appropriate technology, appropriate medicine, and appropriate life-styles all go hand in hand in preserving and enhancing life on our planet.

ARE YOU IMMUNE?
Natural Ways to Build Your Resistance

by William LeSassier

With all the complexities of life, it seems all too easy to become run down. There are, however, many ways to prevent this from taking place.

The body has certain organs that store energy —especially the liver, spleen, and adrenal system. These organs can become depleted. When any one of them becomes too weak, it borrows on other organs and interrelates these imbalances perfectly so the system does not, on the whole, suffer too much. It really pays to do several things when the system is weak: sleep, stay warm, and eat lightly but of nourishing things, preferably with complete amino acid balances. Remember, when the body does not sleep at night the nervous system, lungs, adrenals, and liver all suffer. In order to avoid this we must first understand the healthy immune reaction—what I call attunement.

ATTUNE AND BE IMMUNE

Attunement means acting with your environment, your needs, etc. Whenever you travel, realize that it will take time for the system to adjust to the new environment. Give yourself a day of rest when you arrive and eat sparingly of new foods if you can. This will give you a chance to come into balance with the environment. Some people arrive in Mexico and the very first thing they do is eat hard-to-digest foods and get a case of "Montezuma's Revenge." Others, because of their own ability to flow, have no reaction. A good key to whether or not you travel well (how attuned you are) is to notice how you retain energy. Does your communication from the mouth stop (alienation)? Do you become constipated, or shoulders stiffen? These all come from blocks based on movement, the security or order of one's life being broken. When you are traveling do not set yourself apart. There's an old saying "Commune and become immune." I really believe that a well-tuned body and a little prevention allow one to commune without being affected by negative stimuli.

Immunity can be encouraged by certain herbs. I think traditionally the herbs used most for prevention are herbs that have an aromatic or expulsive property to them. Cayenne, eucalyptus, juniper, garlic, and myrrh are examples of this quality. These herbs contain properties which are antiseptic and warming. They are respected as being protectors in many countries where they grow. Eucalyptus is a well-known influenza preventive and has been helpful in preventing dysentery, pneumonia, distemper in animals, and most respiratory problems. I think that with a little more eucalyptus tea in America most flu could be prevented. Eucalyptus trees purify the air. They have been planted in malaria-ridden swamps and draw up tremendous amounts of water from the roots emitting a natural repellent.

Myrrh in the form of incense has been used to expel negative energies. Myrrh tea taken internally is a most effective antiseptic. However these teas do *not* in themselves influence the system basically like most antiseptic antibacterials. They just stand between an invading field of energy and you. It is good to combine these herbs with deeper acting herbs, in a less symptomatic approach to immunity: chaparral, echinacea, astragalus, horsetail (spring gathered), and crab-apple bark—these teas work more deeply.

Here are some basic immuni-"teas" which have been used successfully. Some of these are composition powders which can be put into 00 capsules (¼ size for children under four, ½ size for children four to seven). Another way of making preparations is to roll the medicines with a small amount of honey and then press into little balls. These can be rolled in powdered herbs and then dried slowly. The trick to making them is to use only a little bit of honey. Another alternative to capsules is rice paper (pure). Herbs can be rolled into this and then swallowed. The paper is just roughage. Up to five caps a day can be taken safely.

INTESTINAL PREVENTIVE

Equal parts of:
  goldenseal
  asafetida powder
  myrrh
  colonsonia
  cascara sagrada
  chaparral

INFLUENZA PREVENTIVE

Equal parts of:
  myrrh
  juniper berries
  calendula flowers
  eucalyptus
  astragalus (Chinese herb)
  echinacea

GENERAL PREVENTIVE

Equal parts of:
  myrrh
  crab-apple bark
  astragalus
  horsetail
  echinacea

These blends can also be made into teas, if you don't like taking capsules. Several cups (one teaspoon herb to one cup water) can be taken. Always steep aromatic herbs. Seldom boil.

It is actually better to devise a formula that would tend to focus on individual herbs, but these formulas serve the purpose well. Many herbs can be a preventive for a given person.

PREVENTION OF DISEASE BY EATING RIGHT

Both the B complex and vitamin A form a basis for prevention. Green leafy foods, unless suspect, are always best for immunizing. B vitamins can be obtained from many grains, peanuts, seeds, and brewer's yeast (but this can be allergenic).

FOODS WHICH BURDEN THE BODY

Certain foods disperse energy from the organs. Overuse of milk products can weaken the spleen.

Overuse of fried food, greasy foods, weaken the liver and gall bladder. Overuse of stimulants, coffee, maté, and others, weaken the adrenals. A good way to tell how much vitality is present in the adrenals and kidneys is to look under the eyes. Those dark circles are sometimes called adrenal ruts.

REBUILDING GLANDS

To rebuild weak glands, B vitamins, sarsaparilla, licorice, and ginseng can be used. These contain plant ingredients that support adrenal functions. These can be made into a formula such as this:

1 part sarsaparilla
½ part licorice
1 part ginseng
1 part astragalus (or burdock root)

Two cups a day for about a week and a good conscious diet.

I think it is important to note the uselessness of the overkill point of view. Unless the system is seriously depleted or seriously diseased it is not necessary to fill yourself with hundreds of vitamins. Let your system develop its own natural resistance to disease. Someone who has not bothered to develop her or his own immunity system because of parental intervention, antibiotics, etc., should be encouraged to do so. It is not necessary to stamp out germs or kill all the flies in the world. I mentioned earlier one cup of eucalyptus tea is a very likely preventive for flu but twenty cups a day would be overkill and would be destructive. In a crisis, five or six cups might be necessary. Use less of a substance when trying to prevent an illness than when trying to cure one.

Granted, sickness is not pleasant, but try to accept and evaluate your energy. Disease is located in certain parts of the body in accordance with influences from the environment (including inner, local, planetary, etc.). It is foolish to think for a minute that things just happen to you without reason. The only kind of feelings that will arise from this attitude are ones of self-pity. Try to examine why things are the way they are and learn how to better them. Try to see clearly that this is the finest art the eyes will ever know. Because disease is a natural working out and discharge of old energy forms, assist rather than resist.

TOOTH YOGA:
How to Care for Your Teeth

by Jim Hall, D.D.S. and Barbara Salat

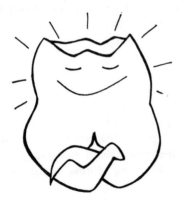

The soft tissues of the mouth reflect the current state of health of the person, and the teeth carry the record and reflect the history of the health. If negative changes are occurring in the mouth, one must recognize this as negative change of the whole.

Negative change may be seen as: decayed and broken teeth—gingival inflammation with reddening, swelling, and bleeding during chewing or tooth brushing—sores on the lips, tongue, or mucous membranes. These changes show an unbalanced state of health.

The mouth is the entrance to the interior of the body, and it reflects the dietary habits and nutritional state most vividly. A regular intake of refined sugars or natural, concentrated sugars such as honey, dates, dried figs, and raisins will affect the whole system starting with destruction of the teeth by decay.

The state of health of the whole body and the separate parts may be seen as an energy state of balance. The energy used in chewing raw foods is beneficial to the stimulation of the muscles, bones, teeth, and periodontal tissues. The energy not used in the chewing of food must be compensated by energy through the arm in tooth brushing to keep tissue health in balance.

If negative change is occurring in the mouth one must evaluate the requirements and put energy into the system by regular, thoughtful brushing of the teeth and gums. Changes in the diet should include less prepared and refined food and more coarse, raw food.

It is important to recognize the sensitivity of the mouth not only to inward flow of nourishment, but to expression—an outward flow of communication so involved with feelings and emotions. The energy state of these feelings and emotions is reflected in the health of the mouth organ. Foods are eaten not only for basic physiologic need, but often to satisfy emotional need.

The mouth is the most active breeding ground for germs of any part of the body. Even the mouth of a healthy person will contain an abundance of germs. This is natural. It is dark, warm, moist, and all too often contains food for bacterial growth—a germ paradise. The main reasons for daily attention to the mouth and teeth are:

1. To remove food . . . even if you chew well and rinse your mouth after eating, tiny particles of food remain. The more food you leave in your mouth to decompose, the greater will be the bacteria population.

2. To disorganize bacterial colonies. It takes twenty-four hours for bacteria to reorganize enough to form plaque (which is just another name for this type of highly organized bacterial colony). These colonies can metabolize carbohydrates left in the mouth, converting them to acids which can irritate gum tissue and dissolve tooth enamel (the hardest substance in the body). This toxic excretion can not only disease your mouth, but can affect the whole body, possibly causing loss of energy or fever. It is actually a low-grade infection. Plaque combines with saliva to form calculus, the hard, off-colored stuff dentists remove when they clean your teeth. Calculus can push back the gums, making disease and decay all the more likely.

3. To stimulate and massage the gums. Regular massage promotes a healthy blood flow which in turn helps prevent disease.

BRUSHING . . .

There are differences of opinion concerning which brushing technique is best. Whatever technique you use, remember to brush thoroughly between the teeth and on the gums. Gently squeeze the bristles into the spaces between the teeth and gums. (Hold the brush on an angle and use a quick vibrating motion to do this.) Watch yourself brush to make sure you get into all the nooks and crannies. You'll enjoy the experience more if you really take interest in what you're doing.

Toothpastes or powders are less important than we have been lead to believe. The good taste or foaminess may make some people enjoy brushing more, but they really are unnecessary. It's the brushing action that does the job. Herbal toothpastes and powders can be beneficial in the treatment of mouth irritations. The most common mixture is equal parts goldenseal and myrrh. To make an herbal toothpaste:

Soak overnight
3 tablespoons Irish Moss in
2 tablespoons water, add
1 tablespoon orris root powder
and thoroughly mix
1 tablespoon comfrey root powder
1 tablespoon myrrh
dash of goldenseal

It won't taste like Crest, but it will have an earthy flavor you can adjust to.

RINSING . . .

Although you can brush your teeth while waiting for a bus, it sometimes just doesn't seem proper to pull out your brush. At times like these, rinse instead and remember to brush and floss later. The vigorous swishing action will dislodge many food particles and temporarily wash away bacterial acids, although it doesn't replace the full treatment.

A warm salt-water rinse will temporarily cut

down the germ population and will make you aware of areas being eaten by decay or disease.

FLOSSING . . .

Bacteria are extremely tiny and can live between the teeth in tiny spaces smaller than a toothbrush bristle. Using dental floss you can disorganize these bacteria, and most of the time even find some food particles that were lodged snugly between the teeth.

Cut off about one foot or more of dental floss. Tie the ends together to make it into a circle. Hold it as shown, wrapping it around each middle finger once to hold it securely.

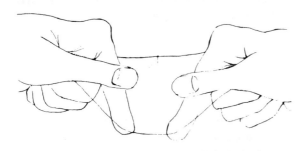

Slide the floss gently between your teeth until it stops above the gums. Scrape the side of one tooth, moving away from the gums, then scrape the other tooth.

It is best to floss when you are relaxed so tension or haste doesn't cause you to force the floss between your teeth, possibly hurting yourself. Get comfortable and watch yourself do it. Imagine all the invisible germ cities you're breaking up.

MOUTH AWARENESS . . .

When was the last time you really looked into your mouth? It is a fascinating organ. It changes daily. You can see your progress as far as mouth care and also note changes due to diet, emotions, and stress.

1. Look closely at each tooth and the gums. Are the teeth stained? Is there food in between? Are the gums a healthy color (color varies with pigmentation). Are they smooth, puffy, or do they have some texture?

2. Feel the teeth and gums. Use your index finger or thumb to help you put the finger on problem areas. Is there pain when brushing or touching? Does the mouth burn or feel hot? Do the teeth feel rough (an indication of calculus build-up)?

3. Smell and taste the mouth. Bad breath and taste can be an indication of poor condition not only in the mouth but in the digestive system as well. And covering it up doesn't really help. Accept whatever you become aware of as your condition right now and look to find and eliminate the cause.

PUTTING ENERGY INTO THE MOUTH . . .

Taking ten minutes per day to do a thorough brushing and flossing puts nurturing, loving energy into your mouth. It's a shame to see people who talk (mouth off) about the need to love oneself become regular dental patients because they just didn't take the time and energy to put self-love to work in the mouth. If you consciously put this kind of good energy into your mouth you'll be repaid with better energy coming out of it—and most likely a set of pearly whites to last a long, long time.

Read—*The Tooth Trip* by Thomas McGuire, D.D.S., Random House, $3.95, for more detailed (although sometimes confusing) information on tooth and mouth care; includes good sections on detecting disease and choosing a good dentist.

THE FINE ART OF SWEATING

by Denni McCarthy

At least twice a week we walk across the field, through the grasses and coyote bush, to our friend's house to sweat together. This has become a beautiful ritual and the whole process an art. My body now expects to sweat, and if I miss a week my system begins to long for it.

The idea of sweating, as a form of bathing, is very old. Romans took regular steam baths in the *calidarium* and we've all heard of the indulgent Turkish baths. The American Indians had sweat lodges which were small stick frame huts covered with a mixture of mud, pine needles, grass, buffalo hides, or even rugs and blankets. They were almost always located by a stream to jump into afterwards and were a place for communal bathing and social gathering. Heated rocks were put into a pot in the center and water thrown on the rocks to create hot vapor. Indian tradition suggested that steam baths chased unwanted spirits from the body. The Finnish sauna differs from these high humidity baths in that the heat is dry, but the effect of sweating is the same.

WHY SWEAT

Sweating expedites the cleansing of toxins. It aids the circulation so that all the organs are stimulated in their activity. The skin, which normally releases about 30 per cent of the body's wastes through perspiration, is our largest eliminative organ. Because of the sedentary nature of many of our life-styles we often neglect and even avoid this natural and important function of the skin. For good health it's essential that we restore and revitalize the cleansing action of the skin. Sweating is a result of "overheating" or fever healing which increases the metabolic processes in our bodies and inhibits the growth of unwanted disease-promoting organisms. They are literally burned up. It is also relaxing to the muscles, effective in dissolving tension, and improves skin tone. A regular program of sweating is an aid in maintaining good health.

WAYS TO SWEAT

I prefer a "dry" sauna as a means of sweating instead of a steam bath with its use of hot vapor. The traditional Finnish sauna is a small wooden room or building with two benches, one above the other. It's heated by a wood stove, gas or electric units on which river bed rocks are placed. During the sauna the rocks are sprinkled with water, producing a fine mist that is quickly absorbed. A sauna is usually 160° to 210° F. and can be taken from ten to thirty minutes. People with heart problems or particularly sensitive systems should sauna with caution. I like to shower to cool off halfway through the sauna.

If a sauna or steam bath is not available we can sweat by soaking in a hot bath for twenty minutes. Afterwards, go into a warm room and wrap up in a large towel or flannel sheet; cover up with lots of blankets. Relax for twenty to thirty minutes and you'll be surprised how much is released.

PREPARING TO SWEAT

It's a good idea not to eat before sweating, since the digestive processes might be disturbed by the radical temperature changes. A hot cup of calendula flower or yarrow flower tea (one teaspoon to one cup boiled water, steeped thirty minutes) can be taken one half hour before sweating. These herbs will help to bring toxins to the surface of the skin and cause the pores to dilate, promoting elimination. A dry-brush massage is excellent to do before bathing. Natural-bristle, long-handled brushes are found at many health-food stores. Rub all over in a vigorous circular motion; the old skin will literally flake off. In Finland they rub each other or themselves with birch twigs both before and during the sauna. This promotes sweating, cleanses the skin, and smells good as well.

IN THE SAUNA OR BATH

Part of the "art" is setting the scene, so we can luxuriate in different aromas, lights, and healing essences. There are many herbs to use for different purposes. One of the first we tried was a

stimulating treat. Make a strong tea of cloves, licorice root, cinnamon, and orange peel—a small handful of each herb steeped forty-five minutes in one quart of boiled water (this is the standard measurement we use for sauna or bath herbs). Strain into the tub or carefully over the hot rocks (the hot steam can burn) and breathe deeply of its invigorating essence. For congestion in the head or sinuses we use eucalyptus or sage. The leaves can be put right on the rocks or in the bath; but we've found a strong tea works the best. To relieve nervous tension (the sweating itself helps) use some chamomile or rosemary in the bath. A headache might be helped by a strong mint brew; all that delicious-smelling steam clears so well. In the bathtub use a few drops of mint oil.

(EDITOR'S NOTE: *Too much mint oil will create a "menthol" effect: cooling rather than warming you when you get out of the bath. A bath in mint oil is a good summertime cooler but it won't help you sweat much. Mint oil in a bath might also be too drying for people with dry skin. So be sure to use just a tiny bit: two or three drops if you're in a bath to sweat.*)

Experiment with different herbs and see what they feel like—bay leaves, lavender flowers, rose petals, and ginger are all good to try.

AFTER SWEATING

After sweating take a cold shower or dip in a pool or stream. This closes the pores and cools the system down. Then RELAX; lie down and do some deep breathing for at least fifteen minutes. We've often found ourselves into yoga (it's so much easier to stretch after sweating) or massage. Oils are wonderful to use now; try some fine almond, apricot, olive, or a special homemade lotion. I like to drink an herbal tea or some pure water after releasing so much of my own water.

When done sweating I feel well cleansed and relaxed. It has been said that everyone looks most beautiful an hour after a sauna. The art is in the ritual, in the time we take to care for ourselves.

The Physiology of Sweat

This entire system is basically a mechanism of temperature control which also happens to include the excretion of waste as a secondary process. Although sweating may be induced by emotional stimuli, such as anxiety or fear, it is primarily induced by an increase in the temperature surrounding the body. When such an increase occurs, the body will respond by sending more blood to the sweat glands and on to the surface of the skin. This blood which comes from deep within the body may measure 99° F., but as it passes near the skin surface, it will release some of this "heat energy" out through the skin and into the droplets of sweat that continually form there. After this release of "heat energy" has taken place, this same blood will return to the body at about 92° F. Meanwhile, the droplet of sweat which absorbs that "heat energy" is being quickly evaporated into the atmosphere carrying the heat with it.

Along with all of this, the constant film of moisture created by the sweat glands forms a layer of insulation that retains the heat we need and keeps out any excess heat. It is able to do this because any heat trying to enter the body must first enter through this layer of sweat which is constantly evaporating.

It should be noted that along with increase in the temperature around us there is a corresponding increase in the stress and strain placed on our circulatory system, and while a healthy, physically fit body should have no problems with this, it would be advisable for anyone with a disorder of the heart or other circulatory organs to check with his or her physician before undertaking the art of sweating. Also, although some fatigue is natural due to the very real expenditure of energy during a sweat session, it is important to remember to *LISTEN TO YOUR BODY* while you are in the sauna. If you feel any exceptional discomfort, dizziness, or extreme weakness realize that your body is trying to tell you that, at least for the moment, it is unable to cope with the extra stress from such high heat.

THE HEALING USES OF WATER

- Water flows life into our bodies, bringing cleansing.
- Bathe in nature's oceans, lakes, and rivers.
- Drink pure water.
- Use cold water for red eyes or nosebleed.
- A warm salt-water rinse through nose cleans out mucus. (This can be done with small flower-watering pitcher.)
- Compresses are folded wet cloths. Hot ones open and stimulate skin action. Cold ones contract and reduce pulse. Alternating ones relieve congestion and pain.
- Try a cold forehead cloth for a headache, a cold spine cloth for nerves.
- An enema quickly cleanses the colon. It is pleasant if approached with a peaceful and positive attitude. Overusing enemas can be harmful.
- A douche can soothe as well as cleanse. Herb teas or yoghurt can be added for extra healing properties.
- Take short, warm baths in herbal water. Eucalyptus, mint, and chamomile are nice.
- Three ways to add bath herbs: 1) Tie in a mesh bag and put in bath. 2) Tie the bag over the faucet. 3) Make a strong tea and add it to the bath.
- End a shower with cold water in order to adapt to temperature change and become "cold" resistant.
- Then wrap up in a blanket, or put on your cotton clothing. Your body will warm the moisture and open your pores to absorb it.
- Hot steam opens pores and draws out toxins.
- Do a sauna, sweat lodge,
- or facial sauna.
- After a sweat or facial, cold water closes pores and stimulates.

MEET YOUR COLON

by William LeSassier

The colon is not easy to clean, rebuild, or even strengthen. The colon responds to many inputs of energy—vertebrae position, the condition of the flora, the mucous membrane, the acid/alkaline balance, parasites, emotions, etc. One must place the organ in an optimum condition to regain balance.

There has been a great controversy over such things as how many bowel movements a person is supposed to have daily. It has been stated that a bowel movement after every meal is considered best. This does indicate great peristalsis. I think elimination does vary greatly from person to person depending on the amount of bulk in the diet, and the quantity as well as the type of food eaten. Most people agree that the morning is the time of greatest elimination. The time of greatest bowel activity is between 5 and 7 A.M. Certainly sleeping too late in the morning will unbalance the colon. However, due to the diversity of colons and opinions it is difficult to establish a standard. It is a matter of individual balance. A healthy colon is responsive to nerve stimuli, and eliminates through peristalsis and gas. (This does not mean fermented "methane-" type gas that everyone dislikes. It means normal, occasional, healthy "wind.)"

CONSTIPATION

Constipation is viewed by many as a cause in itself for disease. This is an incomplete viewpoint. Colon imbalances are symptomatic of imbalances in other systems within the body, and of course do have their effect on other parts of the body. Because it is an organ of elimination as well as nutrition, the colon reflects what other organs are doing or not doing. For example, if the liver is sluggish, the colon will not function properly. A very common cause of constipation which many overlook is excessive urination and insufficient fluids in the body. Any time someone takes diuretics (agents which promote water elimination) without taking in sufficient amounts of fluids, this produces dry stools. Improper food combinations can also produce this dryness by causing so much fermentation that the colon can become hot. The body then sends fluids to the surface of the body to cool the body by evaporation. When there is this kind of dryness in the system, one must use herbs that will expel gas, cool the system, and moisten the stool. A combination of fenugreek, cascara sagrada, and slippery elm will surely relieve the symptoms of dry stools.

The best laxatives to use are actually foods. Carob pods, pecans, agar-agar, tapioca, etc., can be very good. Ripe fruits are all good. Prunes and figs are laxative and can regulate the acid/alkaline balance in the colon. Always soak dried fruit overnight before using it for laxative purposes. Prunes soaked overnight increase the acidity of the colon, expel excess mucus, and eliminate many bacteria, but in excess they can kill the flora and can be irritating to one who has hemorrhoids or is prone to irritation of the mucous lining. Figs are alkaline, emollient, soothing, and cooling to the large intestine. They are bulky, give tone to the colon, increase flora, and are excellent for hemorrhoids.

I don't need to tell many of you about the value of fiber in the diet. Wheat bran, carob, and coarse foods should be part of the diet. The use of fenugreek and wheat sprouts will help keep anyone's colon healthy. The sprouts, eaten when they are seven days old, will aid in the digestion of leftover waste which has caked on to the walls of the colon. These sprouts are cleansers as well as builders.

PREGNANCY

A sidelight for pregnant women: many herbal laxatives are definitely suspect as toxic to fetal activity. Such herbs as mandrake (American), senna, and aloe are to be avoided. Even cascara sagrada, buckthorn, or other rhamnus species are to be avoided, for although they are not directly toxic, they can be irritating.

The safest laxative *tonics* for pregnancy are manna*, butternut bark or root*, flax seed*, slippery elm*, and lemon verbena (very mild). These may be combined with an aromatic such as fennel or anise seed. Take about one tablespoon of the herb to each cup of water. Drink up to three cups daily. However, it is not wise to overdo any kind of laxative unless under the care of a competent herbalist. The herbs I have mentioned here are the least toxic.

HEMORRHOIDS

Hemorrhoids are an engorgement of the blood vessels around the rectal lining. They can become irritated, ulcerated, and can be quite painful. They are due to blocked flow of blood in the veins of the colon. In pregnancy they are common due to pressure on the pelvic floor, which reduces circulation. (This also causes varicose veins.) Cayenne taken internally will stimulate the circulation in the body. The dosage varies greatly, though, from person to person. If you wish to take it, start with small amounts in food or tea, increasing the amount if it does not bother you. Agents like nettles and Irish moss increase blood circulation, which is helpful. Of course, if a person is constipated this should be treated too. Also excess amounts of salt should be avoided as salt creates thick, heavy blood. Heavy uses of curry, black pepper, ginger, and cinnamon can also be irritating to the rectum.

If there is ulceration, irritation, or ineffective elimination, a potato suppository may be useful. Whittle out a piece of raw potato about the size and shape of your little finger. This is inserted overnight and really aids in the healing of hemorrhoids. Slippery elm or flax seed can also be used to soothe this condition. Take them in either tea or suppository form.

DIARRHEA

Diarrhea can be partially caused by a weak spleen. If the spleen is functioning properly, it

* means especially favorable herbs.

will neutralize toxins which enter the system and they will be passed out of the body in an undramatic way. Also, if the intestinal flora is weak, it will be unable to destroy unfriendly flora such as the type often found in spring or winter runoff water. Diarrhea attacks can also be related to the liver.

Whatever the cause, elimination in this way can cause loss of precious electrolytic fluids (digestive waters) which make the absorption of nutrients possible. Debilitation can follow because the body loses its ability to obtain nourishment. To prevent this, drink barley or rice water (boil one cup of rice or barley in eight cups of water for one hour). Cerlery juice, coconut milk, or lime juice can be added to this to cool the colon.

Herbal astringents which aid in the checking of excess discharge may also be useful. Blackberry root*, bush monkey flower, white oak*, bistort root, and cranesbill root have been found effective. Also antiseptic herbs may be useful if the condition has been brought on by amoebic or toxic floral invasions or by parasites.

I urge anyone reading this to realize that your intuition is your guiding force. Sometimes it is necessary to recultivate this in respect to diet and care of the body. But do not mistake "cravings" of all sorts for true intuition. This article was written to promote understanding of the body and not to cause worry over one's condition or diet. I did not go into every aspect because it would have become book-like and hard to digest. Happy floral digestion!

✳✳✳✳✳✳✳✳✳✳✳✳✳✳✳✳✳✳✳✳✳

Healthy flora is essential, as B vitamins are generated by these flora. These friendly flora are also policemen of unfriendly flora, consuming and digesting them as they pass through the system. Here are some things that help create healthy flora: kefir, yoghurt, miso, nuts and seeds (peanuts, almonds, and sesame seeds in particular). Of course a good diet will help maintain healthy flora.

Here are some things which weaken flora: excessive use of garlic (this varies from individual to individual), goldenseal over three double-0 capsules a day (unless under a physician's specific care), enemas in excess, colonics, antibiotics, and, of course, diarrhea attacks. You must re-establish healthy flora through proper diet after heavy cleansing of the colon.

✳✳✳✳✳✳✳✳✳✳✳✳✳✳✳✳✳✳✳✳✳

GETTING INTO FOOT MASSAGE

by David Copperfield

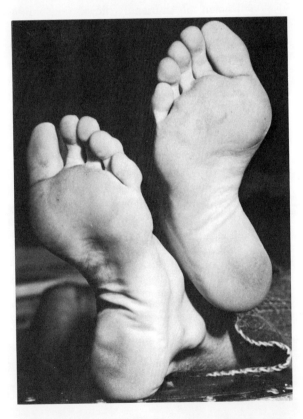

Dr. William F. Fitzgerald discovered that pressure on certain reflex points could bring about the normal functioning of specific organs or areas in the body, no matter how remote from that area the reflex point was. He brought this discovery to the medical world in 1913. Since then, many people have studied and expanded upon this theory.

Reflexology is a scientific technique of massage that has a definite effect on the normal functioning of all parts of the body. There are nerve endings in the feet from every part of the body. These nerves relay conditions in the body. Congestion, toxicity, lowered vitality in any organ will relay as soreness in the related area of the foot. Healthiness will relay as a pleasurable sensation.

Here is a simple technique of foot massage that is good to give and good to receive. It doesn't pretend to be a cure system. It's a general tonic for the body that anyone can give anyone. When received one, two, or three times a week, it will improve your health and vitality. Foot massage is a wonderful way to get to know someone and is lots of fun at parties. Any number of people can form a circle to give and receive foot massages at the same time; groups of four make for good conversation. It isn't necessary to remember all the parts of this technique, or to keep them in the same order. Just allow love and good energy to flow through your hands.

Start by massaging the calf muscle (1) toward

the ankle. Gently massage the ankle and top of the foot (2). Then, placing your thumbs across each other on the bottom of the foot and your fingers interlaced on top, begin an outward motion with the thumbs (3). Work your way from

Hold each point three seconds and move about ¾ inch between "points." If you find some sensitive areas, remember to come back to those later.

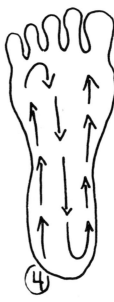

Using both thumbs, work the area below the toes thoroughly (5). Rub across, up and down, and into the cracks between the bones—sometimes this area is sensitive, so get into it slowly.

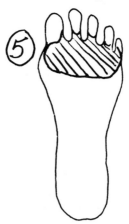

the toes to the heel. Repeat that three times. Now you'll feel "acquainted" with the foot you're working on. Tell your friend you want to use a pressure that "hurts good," so you're asking for assistance and feedback. Using just one thumb or the knuckle of your index finger, begin a deep probe of every inch of the bottom of the foot. Start from the corner of the heel (4) on the little toe side and move up to the little toe, across to the middle, and down to the center of the heel, across and up the instep to below the big toe.

Next, starting with the big toe (6), rotate each toe three times one way and three times the other, wiggle it sideways too, and, finally, give it a little tug. Now massage the areas around the anklebones and Achilles' tendon, using the fingers and thumbs. Massage the area of the top of the foot with your thumb. Get in between the bones and make it "hurt good."

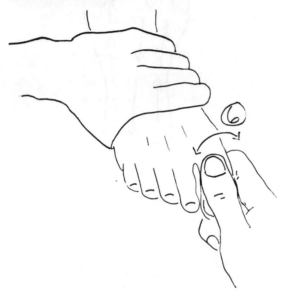

Return to the sensitive areas on the bottom of the foot and, using the ball of the thumb, rotate and press deeply for a few seconds on each area. Now if you want a relaxing finale, softly go over the whole foot, smoothing away tension. Then put the foot down and go on to the other one. If you want an energizing ending, slap the bottom of the foot briskly before starting on the other one.

Caution: Don't push too hard on many places as this can cause too much of a cleansing reaction in the related organs. Gradualness is the key.

If you'd like to learn how to work on specific ailments through reflexology, you'll enjoy *Helping Yourself with Foot Reflexology* by Mildred Carter, Parker Publishing Co., Inc., West Nyack, New York, $2.45.

SHIATSU FOR EVERYBODY

by David Copperfield

Here is a simple massage technique that anyone can learn and use right away. You will be surprised at how much help it will provide for the receiver *and* for yourself. This "Shiatsu for everybody" technique is simplified from more complex techniques you can learn later if you wish.

With your thumbs you will be applying deep pressure along many of the acupuncture meridians

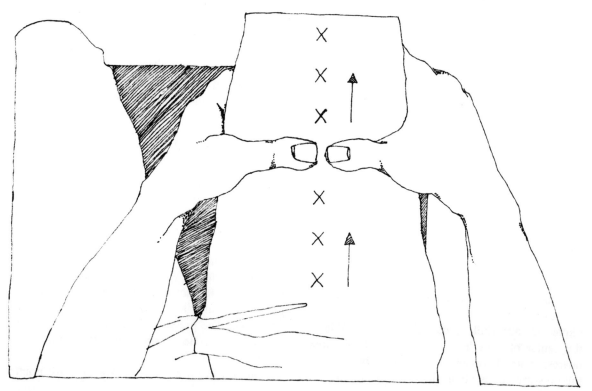

Illustration #1

(energy pathways) thereby benefiting muscles, nerves, and meridians at the same time.

Start right now by placing your thumbs tip to tip (as in illustration ※1) and press on your own upper leg. Allow the thumbs to bend back at the joint (※2). Lean forward, applying more pres-

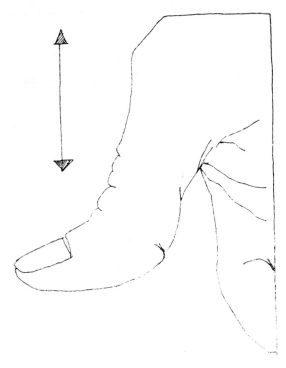

Illustration ※2

sure, and breathe out. Lean back, releasing the pressure, and inhale. Now use this same technique for your whole upper leg. Start on a line in the center of your leg and move from the area nearest your abdomen out to your knee. Space the pressure points about the width of the thumb.

Shiatsu is Japanese finger-pressure therapy using the acupuncture points. Instead of needles, pressure, primarily with the thumbs, is applied to crucial points on the body. Shiatsu treatment brings you relaxation, energy, and mental clarity. It's also a safe home remedy for minor aches and pains associated with tension—headache, backache, stiff neck, insomnia, etc. While practicing Shiatsu, you learn the art of meditative activity, centering, balance, and co-ordination of mind, body, and breathing.

Remember to keep wrists arched, thumbs bent back yet relaxed, breathing out as you lean forward and press down, breathing in as you back off. That's Shiatsu! If you feel you've got it, let's go on.

Choose a quiet place where you won't be interrupted. Have your friend lie face down on a comfortable but firm surface (a mat or folded blanket on a floor is good). Make sure there is plenty of room all around for you to move (perhaps three feet in all directions). Walk over to your friend's right shoulder and kneel on your left knee, keeping your right foot on the floor. Tell him/her to breath with the massage, breathing out with the pressure and in with the release. As tension mounts, your friend should imagine "breathing the tension out with the breath." Ask your friend to let you know if you are pressing too hard or too soft. Let him/her know that the pressure should "hurt good" but not go much beyond that. The pressure should be between pleasure and pain. Be sensitive and stay attuned to what your friend is feeling.

You will begin a series of five pressure points

starting from the right shoulder and continuing down to the bottom of the shoulder blade. The points should be about one inch on your side of the spine. With elbows just a little out, lean forward on your knee, letting your weight rest on your thumbs. Breathe out as you do this. When it's time to breathe in, bring your body weight back. Move your thumbs to the second point, breathe out, and lean forward into your thumbs again. Let slow smooth breathing be your pacing guide. Stay loose and relaxed as your own tension will have an adverse effect on the person being massaged. Rock forward and back smoothly—going forward slowly so that the pressure builds gradually and backing off just as evenly.

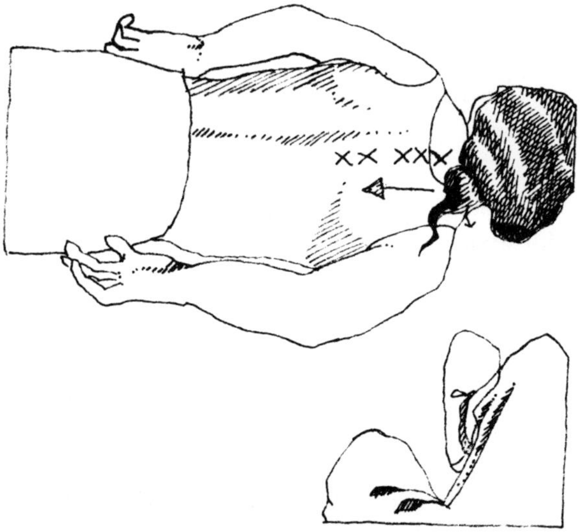

times. Were your elbows out a bit? Did you breathe *out* as you applied pressure and *in* as you retracted? Did you keep your thumbs flat to the first joint? Did you let your body weight do the work?

Now move your knee to a point beside the right buttocks and face the same direction as your friend. Start again with point number 1 just below the right shoulder blade. Your left thumb should just be able to feel the spinal column to the left as you come down the back to point number 8, which is on the edge of the pelvic bone. Repeat the right points two more times for a total of three times. From now on all sets of points should be treated this way (i.e., three times for each set, then on to the next set).

Illustration #3

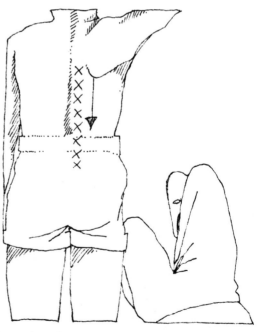

As soon as you reach the fifth point start over on point number 1, repeating all five points. Then repeat all five points again for a total of three

Illustration #4

Move your knee down beside his/her knee and press three points along the edge of the pelvic bone. The third one requires some side pressure. Start on the edge of the pelvic bone and slide into the fleshy area of the back (and side) immediately above the bone. (Repeat three times.)

Feel the spinal area between the pelvic bone and the tail bone. There is just enough room for three points. Do these points three times and don't forget about breathing slowly and evenly.

Do a diagonal of four points across the buttocks three times. Keep your thumbs like this:

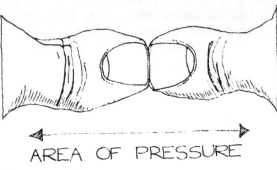

AREA OF PRESSURE

Illustration #6

Your thumbs are like two spatulas that cover a wide area.

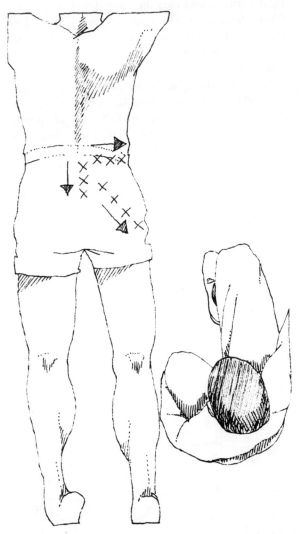

Illustration #5

Now move your left knee all the way down by your friend's ankle. Press ten points along the center of the upper leg starting just under the buttocks and stopping just above the knee. (*Do not* press on the back of the knee.) Smoothly and with little effort rock back and forth on your pivot. (Repeat three times.)

Move your knee to a foot or so below your friend's foot and do eight points along the center of the calf from below the knee to above the heel. (Repeat three times.)

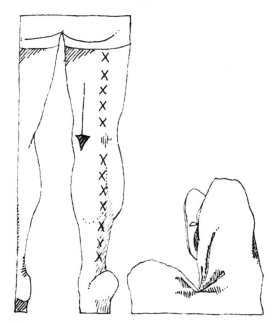

Illustration #7

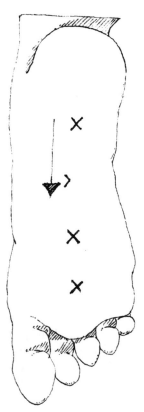

Illustration #8

Now press four points on the bottom of the foot starting just below the heel and stopping just above the toes. (Repeat three times.)

Imagine the flow of energy you have stimulated. See it running from the shoulders down to the foot. Rub your hand firmly over the bottom of the foot from heel toward toes and pull that energy off the foot down onto the floor, grounding it there.

You have now completed one half of the treatment. Get up and go around to your friend's left side, and, kneeling with your right knee near his/her left shoulder, do the five points from the shoulder to the bottom of the shoulder blade on the left side of the spine. Continue the points on the left side just as we did the right. If you find an area of tension spend a little more time and concentration there. Keep your back straight and

your energy together. Remember, you are not "doing it" but allowing natural cosmic energy to flow *through* you and into your friend.

Don't forget to ground the energy into the floor as you finish the left foot. Tell your friend to lie quietly for a while before arising. Sit back and feel your own energy now. Often the person massaging will feel relaxed and invigorated as will the friend who received the massage.

This treatment is less than half of a complete Shiatsu treatment and should take about twenty minutes once you know it. It is, in itself, very effective as an energy balancer to help back problems and to relieve tensions. You will be surprised and pleased at the response of friends after receiving the massage—especially one hour later. The steady breathing, exercise, and allowing cosmic energy to flow through you will, in addition, add a great deal to your well-being.

SHIATSU QUESTIONS AND ANSWERS

An interview with Michael Isquick, who teaches Shiatsu at the University of California at San Diego.

1. *What kind of complaints does Shiatsu help the most?*

Shiatsu works as a preventive, taking healthy clients and keeping them healthy. It is especially helpful when there is tension, or when someone has a dragged-out feeling. It helps relaxation and mental clarity and restores a calm flowing energy. It is a good home remedy for headache, minor aches, nervous stomach, and female problems.

2. *Are there counterindications for the use of Shiatsu?*

Don't use Shiatsu for contagious diseases, serious internal disorders of heart, lungs, liver, or kidneys. Don't use Shiatsu where there is a broken bone or where there is a possibility of internal bleeding (example, ulcers). Shiatsu is not appropriate for treatment of cancer. Serious disorders should be taken to a physician.

3. *Can damage be done by pressure?*

Damage is unlikely if you observe certain guidelines:
a. The cardinal principle—the client determines the amount of pain he can take. If the pain turns from a good, dull hurt to a sharp pain, it's too much for that spot.
b. Note above discussion of counterindications, #2.
c. Use lighter pressure for children, and folks over sixty, people with small or brittle bones.

No bruising should occur if these rules are followed.

4. *Why does it hurt? Does it have to hurt?*

There is misunderstanding about what the "hurt" in Shiatsu means. It should be an almost pleasurable release of pressure. If the receiver is in good shape he can take a fairly heavy amount of pressure without much discomfort, but everyone has a few spots that call for moderate or light pressure. After three or four applications this pain should diminish as circulation is restored to that area.

There are several reasons why it hurts. Usually the muscle is tense at that spot; the pain is an indication of excessive muscle tension. Another reason why Shiatsu can give a good hurt is that acupuncture points are located at sensitive spots on the body, such as the sciatic nerve in the buttocks. A third reason is that, according to acupuncture theory, pain on one of the points alongside the spine indicates trouble within an associated internal organ.

5. *How can the client help?*
a. By steady, rhythmic, deep breathing.
b. By meditating on the breath rather than meditating on the discomfort.
c. By relaxing into the pressure.

6. *How would you compare Shiatsu to acupressure, acupuncture, etc.?*

Acupressure can be used as a synonym for Shiatsu. *Shi* means finger, *atsu* means pressure.

Acupressure connotes pressure on the acupuncture points, and Shiatsu literally means finger pressure.

The use of pressure would have predated the use of needles, since you have your hands before you have instruments. In Shiatsu, pressure is applied primarily with the thumbs, but also with the feet, elbows, palms, and heels. Acupuncture uses needles and is best for dealing with problems of the nervous system, such as nerve deafness. Shiatsu is best for treatment of muscular tension. Shiatsu uses more direct treatment. Acupuncture uses more indirect treatment.

The theory and technique of Shiatsu are very different from that of Swedish massage. The massage is based on Western scientific and analytical understanding of the circulatory system and underlying anatomy and physiology. The oriental system is based on Eastern philosophical understandings of the body and energy flow.

7. *What is the best way to study Shiatsu?*

For those interested in treating muscle tension problems, using Shiatsu as a home remedy, the essentials can be learned in a relatively short period of time. If a person were to learn how to work just on the back he/she would have learned much of the practical aspects. To learn the craft of Shiatsu it is necessary to find a competent teacher. Boston, New York, and San Francisco seem to be main sources of teachers. In New York, for example, there is the Shiatsu Education Center directed by Wataru Ohashi.

AN INTRODUCTION TO HOMEOPATHY

by David Debus

ho-me-op'a-thy, n. [*Gr.* homoiopatheia, *from* homoiopathes *having like feeling or affections;* homoios, *like, similar, and* pathos, *feeling, suffering.*] *The doctrine or theory of curing diseases with very minute doses of medicine which in a healthy person would produce a condition like that of the disease treated.*

Look for the *Physician's Desk Reference* for this year and read the entry under Thorazine. Lots of side effects, huh? Now sample a few other entries, perhaps drugs you have heard about, or have at one time used yourself.

In many countries of the world, homeopathic physicians select remedies for acute or chronic conditions, and sometimes for minor irritations. The reaction of the organism to the totality of the effects is called "provings." These are not like "side effects," in that they can be stopped immediately by the appropriate counterremedy. But when a homeopathic remedy has been correctly applied to a person with a certain constellation of symptoms, there is a cure, rather than a "proving."

In the United States homeopathy is barely known, while for over a century every continent except North America has had a fair percentage of homeopathic physicians. The "lower potencies" of homeopathic remedies are used by the lay practitioner for self and family in simple cases. In the United States homeopathic physicians numbered up to one third the total number of M.D.s at the turn of the century. In the 1920s a combination of forces caused the closing of homeopathic schools and the discrediting of homeopathy. Homeopathy was discounted as a "cult." For more on this, read *The Case for Unorthodox Medicine,* by Brian Inglis.

THE LAW OF SIMILARS

As George Vithoulkas, in *Homeopathy— Medicine of the New Man,* says, homeopathy is a scientific system of medicine, based on principles and procedures which have not changed much since Samuel Hahnemann in the early nineteenth century confirmed Hippocrates' (300 B.C.) Law of Similars. He generalized the law which Hippocrates applied only selectively, and he structured its application. The Law of Similars says that like cures like. This is not fighting fire with fire exactly, nor is it like an inoculation. It follows the Arndt-Schultz Law, accepted generally by people of many medical viewpoints, which states that a large amount of some substance has a different effect from a small amount. Hahnemann found that a very small amount had the effect of curing symptoms brought on by the large amount. A simple example is homeopathic coffee, *Coffea cruda,* which cures that increased sensitiveness, tight head pain, excessive wakefulness, etc., that large amounts of coffee cause. Each remedy is "proved" by observing what it does to a wide range of healthy people. These healthy people briefly exhibit symptoms which the remedy can cure.

(EDITOR'S NOTE: *It's interesting to realize that homeopathy is safe enough to test on people and that this human testing may be far more accurate for us humans than studies done on other animals, i.e., rats and dogs.*)

THE LAYMAN'S USE OF HOMEOPATHY

Now I'm one of those types who sit a lot, and don't exercise as they should, who have a strong tendency toward tobacco, coffee, and wine. There are other broad descriptions of myself I could offer as well, which are perfectly described under *Nux vomica* in the homeopath's *Materia Medica* (Boericke, 9th edition). Since homeopathy treats the patient and not the disease, when I have some little ailment for which a number of remedies seem indicated, including *Nux,* I know which one to take. For, yes, I am treating the ailment, but I am also treating myself.

There are certain physical *and mental* signs which tell me it is time to put those little milk-sugar pellets under my tongue and let them dissolve—I don't touch them, for they are very sensitive to influences from heat, odor, touch, etc. I wait half an hour before and half an hour after taking *Nux* or any remedy, before I eat, smoke, or drink anything. The tissues under my tongue absorb that tiny amount of the remedy present in the milk-sugar tablets directly into the blood stream. The milk sugar is a boat in which the extremely minute remedy can ride safely to its destination. Some say it gets to the right destination in the same way that nutrients from our food get to the right cells to nourish them.

I've learned to take *Allium cepa* (that is, onion) in homeopathic potency when that sneeze which begins a cold occurs. I take *Aconite* for certain kinds of anxieties, or when I have certain cold symptoms.

HOMEOPATHIC FLUORIDE

Because of the water fluoridation controversy, I looked up the entry in the *Materia Medica* under *Calcarea fluorica.* It escaped my understanding why a substance classified as a class-A poison would be put into our water supply. I found an awful portrait of that poison: knots in the female breast; goiter; depression, fear of financial ruin; blood tumors in the newborn; ulcers on the scalp; jawbone swelling; sore or hoarse throat; chronic lumbago—and much more. While I wondered why a poison was proposed for our water supply, I know what to take if some portrait of these symptoms showed up in my life: a few homeopathic doses of the same stuff.

HOW ARE THE REMEDIES PRESCRIBED?

But it is not fair to oversimplify the difficulty of prescribing homeopathic remedies properly. In fact, that's one of the main drawbacks for a physician interested in exploring homeopathy—there is a lot of memory work involved. While some things are generally useful for many people (for instance, homeopathic doses of *Sepia* and *Belladonna* treat the physical-mental problems common to some before and during difficult menstruation), other remedies are more difficult to choose among.

I have found that I needed to know a lot about my physical-mental make-up before I used the right remedy for a particular headache. But that is because, while aspirin removes symptoms ("fast, fast, fast relief"), the right homeopathic remedy, according to the books I've read, treats the underlying condition which produces my headache; that right remedy may also cure a liver imbalance, a craving for sweets, or a hangover. I must have a fair idea of how the headache started, whether it moves about and in what direction, what sort of pain it is, and whether it is accompanied by excitement, cold hands, diarrhea, constipation, faintness, or anything else.

There really are no shortcuts to the memorizing of thousands of remedies with tens of thousands of little quirks, but it is possible to acquire a beginner's knowledge of some of the remedies which work for specific things. In *Homeopathy for the First-Aider,* by Dr. Dorothy Shepherd, for instance, there are a number of remedies given for pain, aches, bruises, wounds, poisons, boils, etc. She begins her section on pain: "Pain from mental or physical shock is relieved rapidly by *Arnica.* . . ." I should say so! And it also helps me out when I overdo exercises, or when my voice is weak from too much singing. I read about its use for stroke patients, and wonder whether an orthodox physician might want to read up on *Arnica* and give it a try in such a case.

HOW ARE THE REMEDIES MADE?

Homeopathic remedies are made with a tiny amount of the substance which is agitated or spun in a solution of water and alcohol called a "solvent." This motion breaks the intermolecular energies of the substance down, releasing them. If matter is crystallized energy, perhaps this action releases the energy in particular substances, called "dynamic energy" of the remedy. One drop from the "mother tincture" is put with nine drops of the solvent. This is "potentized" by shaking, and one drop of the resulting solution is put with nine drops of solvent. The procedure is repeated a third time to produce what is called the "third decimal" or "3x." It is sprayed on milk sugar, which is formed into pellets. It is a fairly low potency, appropriate for home use. The higher potencies, 100x, 200x (much smaller amounts, and although it sounds paradoxical, much more potent) are preferred for long-standing or acute and dangerous conditions. These are best left to the experienced homeopathic physician to prescribe.

I have avoided some theoretical differences among homeopaths in order to make the main points clear: Treat the person and not the disease; homeopathy is scientific in method and treatment; and the Law of Similars—like cures like. On these basic notions, all homeopaths, so far as I know, agree.

WHERE ARE SUCH PHYSICIANS?

Write to the Homeopathic Information Service of the American Institute for Homeopathy, 66 East Eighty-third Street, New York, New York 10028 for more information.

(For information on professional courses in

homeopathy for M.D.s, publications, and information, write to:

National Center for Homeopathy
6231 Leesburg Pike
Falls Church, Virginia 22044)

BIBLIOGRAPHY

Boericke, William, M.D. *Materia Medica, with Repertory* (9th ed.). Philadelphia: Boericke and Runyon. First printed 1927.

Coulter, Harris L., Ph.D. *Homeopathic Medicine.* Washington, D.C.: American Foundation for Homeopathy, paperback, 1972.

Shepherd, Dorothy, Dr. *Homeopathy for the First-Aider.* Rustington, Sussex, England: Health Science Press, paperback, 1972 edition.

Vithoulkas, George. *Homeopathy—Medicine of the New Man.* San Francisco: Kouros Books, 1971. It has been recently reprinted; paperback.

YOU CAN IMPROVE YOUR VISION

By Jerrian J. Taber

Yes, you can improve your vision if you want to. But you say, "How can this be?" You have always been told that once your vision deteriorates there is nothing that can be done to reverse the process. It makes no logical sense that if nature with all of her rejuvenating qualities has made allowances for the human body to heal and mend itself that she would have stopped with the organs of the eyes. The truth is that the process of deterioration can be reversed and is reversed by those who are willing to re-educate themselves by a system of vision training. The particular system of vision training I use was developed around the turn of the century by Dr. William H. Bates, an ophthalmologist.

Dr. Bates was an orthodox ophthalmologist—soundly scientific and considered an authority by members of his profession. In 1886 he introduced a new operation for relief of persistent deafness consisting of incising the eardrum membrane, an operation still in use today. In 1894, as a research physician, he discovered the astringent and hemostatic properties of the aqueous extract of the suprarenal capsule, later commercialized as adrenalin.

DR. BATES'S SEARCH FOR THE CAUSE OF POOR VISION

Dr. Bates was not satisfied with the prevailing theory of accommodation (how the eye focuses).

The prevailing theory of accommodation was, and still is, that the curvature of the lens of the eye is the only part responsible for accommodation and that it is its inflexibility that causes failing sight. This happens to a large number of the population around the age of forty and is commonly called "old age sight," presbyopia, or farsightedness. But this term doesn't apply to younger children who certainly cannot fall into this category, or anyone who has not reached age forty. For this we are told that the eyes are abnormally long, or in other words, it is a structural problem of the eyeball. This is commonly called myopia or nearsightedness. This still does not account for the fact that before the person had eye problems there was no structural problem.

For years Dr. Bates felt there was something wrong about the procedure of prescribing glasses to patients who came to him about their eyes. "Why," he asked, "if glasses are correct, must they be strengthened continually because the eyes, under their influence, had weakened? Logically, if a medicine is good, the dose should be weakened as the patient grows stronger."

Dr. Bates gave up his lucrative practice and went into the laboratory at Columbia University to study eyes as they had never been studied before. Disregarding all he had learned in textbooks, he experimented on eyes with an open mind. He ran experiments on animals and examined thousands of pairs of eyes. He never restricted himself to the usual eye examination room, but carried his retinoscope with him, inspecting the refractive state of eyes of both people and animals in many different situations. He refracted eyes of people when they were happy and sad, angry and afraid. Much of this time was spent with children, attempting to discover the cause of eye disorders. His retinoscopic findings indicated that the refractive state of the eye was not the static condition textbooks reported, but varied tremendously with the emotional state. He published an account of a little girl who developed temporary myopia when she lied to him. This fact seemed very significant to him as it was consistent with other findings of myopia, that people tend to become myopic when apprehensive. Therefore Dr. Bates found that the eye is never constantly the same, that refractive error changes momentarily, that mental strain and tension increased it and relaxation decreased it. His conclusions were that imperfect sight was not possible without first a mental strain; that eyes are resistant to what happens from the exterior; that they could mend rapidly from scratches, bumps, and even burns, but could be blinded by mental strain.

HOW THE EYE FOCUSES

His laboratory experiments included the discovery of the function of the six extrinsic (outer) muscles. There are four recti muscles: one on top of the eye, one on the bottom of the eye, and one on each side of the eye. Two muscles belt the eye around the middle and are called oblique muscles. In the body there are two types of muscles, striated (striped) and smooth. The striated muscles are conscious command or voluntary muscles. You decide to take action and do, such as move your head, move your hand, or walk. The

smooth muscles constitute such muscles as the heart, lungs, stomach, and digestive organs. These are involuntary muscles and function unconsciously. You don't tell your stomach to digest your food, it just functions upon ingestion of food. Dr. Bates discovered that the extrinsic muscles (four recti muscles and two oblique muscles) are striated voluntary except where they are attached to the sclera or white part of the eye. Here they become smooth. The striated portion of the recti muscles are voluntary and move the eye up and down and side to side. The striated portion of the oblique muscles helps to rotate the eye. The smooth portion is responsible for accommodation (focus). The recti muscles flatten the eye, shortening the focal length from front to back for distant seeing. The oblique muscles squeeze the eye long, lengthening the focal length for near seeing. All this occurs because muscles only pull (or contract) and relax. When the recti muscles pull to flatten the eye for distant seeing, the oblique muscles have to relax, allowing this to occur. The reverse is true when a person wants to

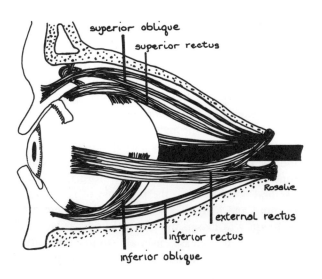

superior oblique
superior rectus
Rosalie
external rectus
inferior rectus
inferior oblique

focus on something at the near point. The recti muscles have to relax, allowing the obliques to squeeze the eye long from front to back. The lens of the eye works in conjunction with the extrinsic muscles. The lens is attached by the cilliary muscles and is thinner when the eye is flattened and contracts (gets thicker) when the eye is elongated or lengthened. In other words, correct focus depends on proper elongation. The eyes works exactly like a camera; it has to change in focal length in order to accommodate.

All these muscles have to work in perfect harmony in order to have normal vision. As previously stated, mental tension or strain is the cause of imperfect sight. The tension is in the mind first and then manifests in the body, not the other way around. Vision is $9/10$ mental and $1/10$ physical. If the oblique muscles are tense and won't let go, the eye cannot accommodate for distant seeing. If the recti muscles are tight and won't let go, the eye cannot accommodate for near seeing. The degree of tension in either muscle group determines the resulting error of refraction (or how much the eye is out of focus).

LEARNING TO RELAX

A Bates Method vision instructor teaches relaxation and helps the student to re-educate mind and body in good visual habits again. You cannot exercise an involuntary muscle; it first has to be relaxed and through relaxation is allowed to function better. It is only through function that the eye can become stronger and in turn can only function through relaxation. Therefore the Bates Method is based upon the principle of relaxation of mind and body. To accomplish this, there are techniques to loosen the physical body as well as techniques to release mental strain. Memory, imagination, and visualization play an important part in re-establishing eye-mind co-ordination and normal vision.

HOW LIGHT AFFECTS SIGHT

Eyes are the only organs in the body constituted to receive and use light. The *fovea centralis* calls for stimulation by light. This impulse must be responded to or it will perish. Eyes that have plenty of light are strong; those starved for light are weak. Eyes dwelling in darkness where the need for light is prohibited go blind. It is found throughout all nature that the birds, beasts, and fish who live in environments where the light is strongest have the most excellent vision. Moles, earthworms, and fish in the ocean depths where no light penetrates are blind. They are blind because vision for them was an unused, unnecessary thing. Burros that were made to work in coal mines soon lost their vision, which was regained after they were returned to work in sunlit fields.

When sunglasses are worn, man is going against nature and the normal function of his own light receiving organs. Sunglasses weaken the eyes instead of helping them and lead to poorer vision and weaker eyes.

The Bates Method teaches how to accept and receive light safely and easily so one can reverse this process of light sensitivity. Even if a person has normal vision and is sensitive to light, it would be wise to learn these simple techniques to prevent vision problems. Light sensitivity is the first sign of tension in the eyes.

REBUILDING GOOD VISION

Action of the eye in relaxation is the secret of all normal vision. When people with imperfect vision acquire the art of seeing, the organs of vision will tend to rid themselves of their physical defects. Relaxed organs enjoy better circulation than organs wrongly used and under strain. Improved circulation gives an organ the chance to build up resistance, heal its disease, and correct its defects. This accounts for some of the spectacular results this method has had with people whose eyes had been given up as hopeless, such as Aldous Huxley, who wrote a book about his experiences with the Bates Method titled, *The Art of Seeing,* which is available in bookstores. There are numerous other books written about this method. One of the greatest contributions to the Bates Method was made by Margaret D. Corbett. Mrs. Corbett was trained by Dr. Bates before he died. She spent forty years teaching relaxation and developing techniques. In her school in Los Angeles she taught students and she trained teachers in the Bates Method. She has contributed three books on the Bates Method; *How to Improve Your Sight; Help Yourself to Better Sight;* and *Quick Guide to Better Vision.* There is also Dr. Bates's own book available, called *Better Eyesight Without Glasses.*

The Bates techniques are wonderful to know as a preventive for those with normal vision to insure against eye strain and tension. College students and those who use their eyes a lot could benefit greatly. If a person would contact a vision trainer at the very onset of a vision problem, he might prevent the use of glasses entirely.

Jerrian wore glasses for ten years before learning the Bates Method. She enjoyed the training (and the results) so much that she went on to become an instructor. She currently teaches in the San Diego area. For more information about the Bates Method, write to the author at: 11303 Meadow View Road, El Cajon, California 92020. Or call (714) 447-7801 or 440-5224.

NUTRITION AND THE EYES

A good diet including plenty of raw foods and especially sunflower seeds is helpful in improving vision. The eye muscles are hard working muscles and deserve to be fed well. Linda Clark, in her book *Get Well Naturally,* says that people who work under bright lights use more vitamin A than normal. Vitamin A increases the blood supply to the eye, bringing other nutrients to feed it too.

MAYBE YOU CAN DO WITHOUT GLASSES

by Jerrian J. Taber

Vision comes to normal and relaxed eyes as effortlessly as scent to the nostrils, music to the ear, or the touch of velvet to the fingertips. The tension that causes eye strain can be relieved by relaxation. By natural methods, vision can be improved and eyes can become normal and relaxed.

The purpose of the Bates Method is to teach persons with vision defects to use their seeing organs in the right way rather than the wrong way, to get rid of bad habits of improper use, and to restore normal and natural functioning.

Frequently the dividing point between a normal and abnormal pair of eyes is its impulse to blink under a given situation. If the eyes are perfectly normal, they will blink; suppression of the act of blinking shows the tendency for vision to be abnormal.

NOSE DRAWING

Close your eyes and imagine that attached to your nose is a long black felt marking pen. Imagine a large sheet of white poster paper in front of you. Moving your head, draw a nice large circle with your imaginary pen on your imaginary sheet of paper. Then within the circle, draw a plus sign $+$, and when you have gone over it several times, superimpose an X and go over that several times. There are numerous other objects you can draw such as: eights 8 , lazy eights ∞, and if you put the two together you have a four leaf clover.

You can remember the days while in school and you were doing penmanship drills such as: *llll* ; *ffff* ; *ffff* etc. Whatever you choose to draw, always sign your name and put the date at the bottom of your paper.

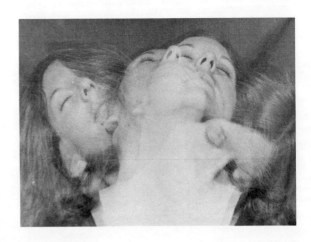

Be sure not to let your mind wander while doing drills. Attend what you are doing because whenever the mind thinks shape or motion and the body does it, the eyes begin their vibrations and better vision results. These drills loosen tensions at the base of the skull, the main nerve center of the body, which is the seat of all tensions.

THE FINGER SWING

While still in bed, close your eyes, put the index finger a short distance from your nose, approximately 2½–3 inches. Pivot the head from shoulder to shoulder on the pillow, whatever your pillow will allow, imagining where the finger is, as the finger and the face pass each other. Now open your eyes and continue the swing from shoulder to shoulder. Your finger will appear to move from ear to ear with a gentle rhythmic motion.

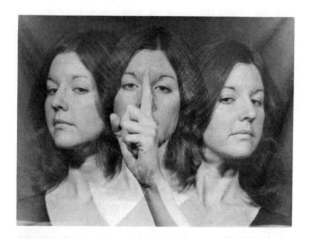

Do not focus on the finger, but let it pass by as your vision sweeps the ceiling, directed only by your nose. Continue alternating between both eyes open and both eyes closed as in the long swing. Do this until the eyes feel loose and easy and you have a good sense of motion.

This particular swing is known for stopping or preventing headaches and can be done anytime during the day while sitting or standing. Be sure the head is pivoted directly above the spine (not slumped). This drill can be used as a first aid against tension.

PALMING

If you are in bed when you palm, tuck a small pillow under each elbow as you lie on your back. It is possible also to palm at a desk or table top by resting the elbows, with or without a small pillow under them on a flat surface before you. Be sure to maintain the straight line of the neck with the spine. Do not bend the head forward. If you find it necessary to lower the head to reach the palms, bend forward from the waist. Palming does little good when the body is rigid and ill at ease.

Form the hand into a hollow cup and place the cupped palm over the eye. The bony part of the hand just above the wrist will rest on the cheekbone. With the fingers crossed over the top of the

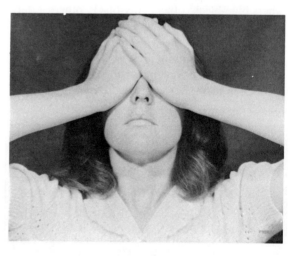

nose, resting lightly against the forehead, you will find that the cup of the hand will fit nicely over the orbit on the eye, the pad of the knuckles resting on the bony structure of the brows. All the light will be excluded when you find the perfect place for your hands. Before placing the hands, lift the brows, then hold them with the hands so that the weight of the brows is lifted from the eyes. This will be of benefit to the nerves around the eyes. Put each hand in place, crossing the fingers over the forehead. Open the eyes only to be sure all the light is excluded, then close them lightly for the rest of your palming period. If when you start a bit of light seems to creep in around the nose area, shift your hands around a little and you will soon find the perfect position for you, and be able to quickly find the correct position again.

When palming is entirely successful, the eyes will experience a sensation of velvety blackness, free from color or grayness or images. The degree of blackness that you obtain is like a steam gauge on an engine. It indicates the degree of relaxation you have achieved. So long as a tension exists you will not see black. Some people see colors, others blue-black, others gray-black, others a dark background, on which there are lighter patches.

As all light has been excluded from the eyes, these colors are simply illusions. They are caused by strain and tension. In other words, you really *do not* see them, however vivid they may appear.

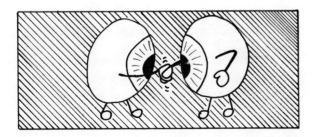

Ignore them, as they will disappear as you attain mental relaxation. Palming is more a mental technique than a physical technique. Its success depends on your own mental habits. If you do experience some difficulty at first, be patient with yourself and do not give up. You will become better with practice.

It is important at this point to be sure that you have a clear understanding of what you are trying to accomplish. The purpose of palming is to achieve mental relaxation. This mental relaxation is not achieved by *trying* to see black. This implies strain and effort. To achieve complete mental relaxation, eliminate all extraneous thoughts from your mind, not by attempting to empty the mind, but by directing it. The best way to accomplish this is to think of pleasant happy memories. Perhaps it is a scene on a river, floating past the shore in a boat; perhaps a skiing trip, soaring down the slope of a mountain; perhaps a quiet hour in a garden, watching large fluffy white clouds floating by against a beautiful blue sky. By conjuring up mental pictures of pleasant past memories you are directing your mind to one thing best and one thing at a time.

Whatever the scene you choose to recall, do not strain to remember it. Let the picture drift through your mind. Fill in the details one by one; the twisted branch of a tree that hung over the river, the soaring motion of a bird in flight, the lovely rhythm of a child's body as it ran.

In your memory pictures, remember the feel of things, such as the warm sand trickling through your fingers, or the rough shell of a peanut. Remember the smell of the ocean or the mountain air. Remember the sound of the gulls, the waves, singing birds, a darting gray squirrel. Be sure your memories are active and in motion. Start to become aware of how much motion is around you all day as you do your daily tasks.

The eyes *do not see;* they merely record sense impressions, which are then used by the mind to see with. This fact has been recognized by philosophers from at least the fifth century B.C. A newborn baby has well-developed eyes and a rudimentary mind. Consequently, it does not see objects in the outside world; it is merely aware of patches of color. In time the baby learns to interpret those colored patches as the appearances of objects external to itself; and the capacity to interpret correctly and to see accurately goes on increasingly with the accumulation of experience in the memory.

Oculists and optometrists are interested primarily in the shape of the eyes at the moment of their examination. They almost never inquire how those eyes (much less the seeing mind) are being used, or what may be the effect upon vision of proper eye use on the one hand, improper use on the other. All they do is to prescribe artificial lenses, which are to defective eyes what crutches are to defective legs. These eye crutches mechanically neutralize the symptoms of defective vision; *they do not remove the cause.*

In the Bates-Corbett Method of visual re-education, the mental side of seeing is taken fully into account, and the main stress is laid, not on the shape of the physical organs at the time of examination, but on the functioning of the eyes and mind during ordinary circumstances of everyday life.

As with all other forms of education, it is difficult for people suffering from serious defects to acquire proper habits of use without the aid of a competent teacher. But there are certain simple techniques which can easily be learned without a teacher's help. Practicing these techniques can do much to relieve the discomfort so often associated with defective vision, and to improve the capacity for seeing, sometimes to a marked extent. In what follows, I shall attempt to describe some of these relaxation techniques.

MOTION IS LIFE!

First of all I would like to explain to you a little about motion. Motion is fundamental to all living things. Even the tiniest cell contracts and expands. Cells in our body are ever being replaced by new ones. Plants are ever growing and expanding. Without motion living things wither and die. So it is with vision; the ocular muscles can become tense and immobile due to strain caused by our habits and emotions. Thank goodness, nature has not left us stranded. If muscles can tense, they can loosen and motion can be regained.

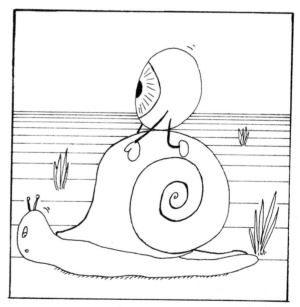

SWING TO RELAX

The following is called the long swing or the elephant swing. The purpose of the swing is to create a sense of motion, or an illusion of motion. The long swing is not a seeing drill but a general body loosener, relaxing and sending ease throughout the entire body.

To do the long swing, stand with the feet about one foot apart, turn the body to the right—at the same time lifting the heel of the left foot. Do not move the head or eyes but let them follow the turn of your body. Now place the left heel on the floor, turn the body to the left, raising the heel of the right foot; alternate. Let the arms hang limply from loose shoulders letting the momentum of the swing lift and swing them free as you turn from side to side. Count out loud rhythmically in tempo with the swing. This is of most importance because when speaking or singing it is impossible for you to hold your breath. Breath holding is a companion of tension. Deep rhythmic breathing is most necessary for relaxation and good vision. Do not think of the swing as an exercise. Think of it as a pleasant surrender to rhythm, such as you would give to a waltz. It is very relaxing to listen to enjoyable music and swing, preferably waltz tempo.

Be sure that the neck, shoulder, and chest muscles are loose and at ease. Swing all of you to one side, then to the other. This creates a half circle or a turn of 180 degrees. Up to the count of seventy-five you are developing the relaxation you need. From seventy-five to one hundred and fifty your body experiences full release of nerves and muscles, every vertebra being loosened, all the inner organs being relaxed. Unknown to the owner, the eyes began to shift with their many involuntary natural vibrations which bring improved vision. Pay no attention to your eyes; you will not be able to feel the involuntary motion. You will know when it is occurring because the entire room will start slipping past you in the opposite direction, as if you were on a merry-go-round traveling back and forth. You leave one side, you leave the other side. Do you get the feeling the room is sliding past? Rest your visual attention approximately furniture height. Do five to ten swings with your eyes open, then close and remember the room slipping by for the same amount of swings. Alternate between open and closed, always remembering what you saw with your eyes open (the room slipping past).

The long swing helps to relax the eyes before sleeping.

RELIEF FOR SORE EYES

If your eyes feel as though you would like to rub them, the following is a great aid. Squeezing the eyelids tightly shut for a second or two, then open them as wide as possible. Repeat this four or five times, or until relief is felt. The pressure of the eyelids gives the eyeballs a thorough massaging, far better than with the hands. This also speeds the circulation through the eyeballs and strengthens the blinking muscles.

MORNING EXERCISES

As discussed earlier, normal seeing depends on mobility of the attention and of the eyes. To restore this mobility, the following simple techniques are to be practiced upon first awakening from sleep, while still in bed.

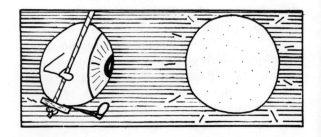

STRETCH AND YAWN

First stretch the entire body out and let go. Find every muscle you can and tighten it, then let go. Yawn and take some deep breaths, then be sure to let all the air out. Repeat this several times. Wiggle your body like a fish. This helps to wake the body up for the day's adventures. Rather than getting up bleary-eyed and groggy, start the day bright-eyed.

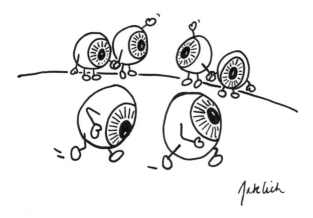

BLINK

Blinking is a quick, light, easy closing and opening of the eye, and it is done intermittently by every normal eye. The rate of blinking varies with people and also varies with the use an eye is put to. You blink more, for instance, when you look at something brilliant than you do when you look at something soft in tone.

Inhale as you do ten quick little butterfly blinks, not hard closings in which your whole face participates, but light, feathery little blinks. Then close the eyes and as you exhale turn your head from side to side, imagining you are blowing soap bubbles from your mouth. Watch them and see them float and dance around. Notice the reflection of the rainbow from them as they float past. Repeat this ten times.

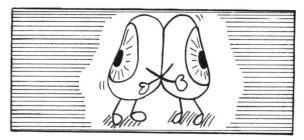

If it is a garden you have remembered in your mind and are visualizing, begin to look at one flower bed, now at one rose bush, and now at a single rose, until you see it clearly and in detail. Be sure your mind does not wander to other subjects, to other pictures, or to other thoughts. Keep your mind in attendance to what you are remembering or visualizing. In visualizing, always select the thing in which you are most interested, because the greater the attention you have bestowed on an object the more perfectly you will remember it, and your visualizing will depend on the sharpness of your memory. If visualizing is difficult, be patient with yourself and pick very simple and familiar objects at first. Do not work at this. Do not concentrate or frown or force yourself grimly to remember. Relax and let the memory come to you.

The following is an example of an excellent mental picture utilizing most of the senses. Notice and become aware of the motion involved.

Visualize yourself lying on the sand. The sun feels warm on your body. There is a soft cool breeze; feel it on your face and body. The smell of the salt water is in the air; take a big breath and remember the smell. You lazily open your eyes (in memory) and look at the water. The ocean is a lovely blue-green, with white waves as they come breaking onto the shore. They break gently at first, then seem to increase in size. Here comes a big one, BOOM! it hits the shore. It recedes with a swish, leaving the wet sand in its wake, with bits of kelp and shell and tiny bugs. You watch this movement for a moment then let your eyes drift out over the water. A sail boat is there and you watch it go on and out toward the horizon where the water is a soft lavender, blending into the sky. Two gulls nearby attract your attention and you watch them floating over a bit of fish. One makes off with it and you see the other soaring over the water, darting up and down until he, too, flies away.

Always take your mental pictures from things you enjoy; otherwise they would not bring relaxation, but would only add to the tension. Learn to love your palming time in order to receive the maximum results. Palm as often as possible, morning and evening as minimums, ten to fifteen minutes at a time, longer if possible. You cannot palm too long. It is very beneficial, so look for opportunities during your day to palm or do some of the above drills as your profession allows.

I have received many letters from all over the United States from those expressing the desire for normal vision and wanting to know the name of a teacher in their area. Unfortunately most of the teachers are concentrated in Southern California, as Mrs. Corbett's school was located in the Los Angeles area. There is a great need for teachers all over the United States. I have been training teachers for this purpose. I am looking for qualified people to come to San Diego for six months to take the bulk of their training and finish at home the following six months. Send me a résumé of your background and interests if you are interested in teacher's training.

Jerrian J. Taber Studio
11303 Meadow View Road
El Cajon, California 92020

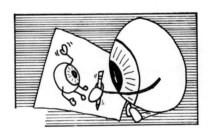

NATURAL FIRST AID FOR MINOR INJURIES

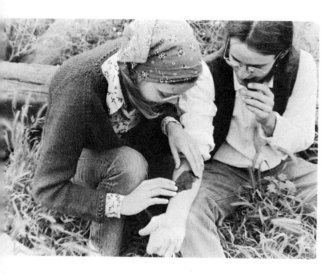

These are some suggestions for what to do in case of minor injuries while camping.

1. *Keep your act clean*—This is more important than it seems at face value. When you are hiking or generally exercising more than usual, you can expect to sweat more. In order to keep the elimination through your skin happening and keep other critters from living off of you, wash off daily, rinse out your socks (especially), and check yourself and your partner for ticks. In washing you not only become aware of ticks and generally get more comfortable, you also find those stiff hiking muscles which a little gentle massage and some eucalyptus oil, if you have it, will take care of. Washing can be done in a surprisingly small amount of water too. For merely removing excess dust and sweat, soap isn't necessary. A good thick washcloth or a loofa sponge would be helpful though, and light. Liquid biodegradable soap is easy to carry and versatile, if you feel you need it. *Wash all injuries thoroughly.* Use your drinking water or boil water from creeks, etc., if you suspect any form of contamination. This will help the body attend to healing the wound rather than having to fight infection.

2. *Rest when you're tired*—There's nothing more satisfying than pushing on to your destination and going beyond your physical barriers. But enough's enough. Injuries such as twisted ankles, etc., are more likely to occur when you are overtired. Be aware of your energy level. Like an animal in nature, the strong, alert, and aware survive.

3. *Be patient and thorough when treating a wound*—First of all take time to stop the sight-seeing and concentrate on healing. Look carefully. See how and why it happened. Look at the extent of the injury and how best you can bring it comfort. Tune in to the environment around you: what can be of use:

plants? charcoal? mud? water? A simple burn, bruise, blister, or sprain can become much more unpleasant than usual if not cared for. When you're camping, these things get exposed to the elements, and the areas affected are often used more than they should be. If handled with patience and awareness, wounds can heal more quickly.

Blisters   Look to the cause. Work boot leather to soften it. Change socks. Broken blisters can become infected in sweaty socks, so get to that blister when you first feel it. Otherwise, it will be more work later. Cold water will help relieve pain and take down the swelling. Some sort of loose padding on it might protect it if it breaks, or cushion it enough to prevent that from happening. Puncture a blister only if absolutely necessary (that is, if you think it will probably break anyway). Do this carefully, using a sterile, sharp tool. Puncture from the side of the blister, and allow the fluid to drain. Apply an antiseptic dressing, and bandage neatly and securely (not too tightly) with a sterile cloth or bandage.

Burns   Protect yourself from the sun. Keep the burned area moist, using water, oil, aloe vera, poultices.

Cuts   Wash the wound. Examine for any particles, etc. Help it to close by applying a plantain poultice. Chew a leaf of plantain to release its juices, then tape or bandage it into place with tape or a clean cloth.

Poison oak, ivy, etc.   Wash with cool water to remove surface oils. Keep internal system flowing with plenty of fluids and light foods. Mud, manzanita, and mugwort have all been useful. Use "itch" energy in other, more constructive ways. Baking soda also makes a good itch-relieving poultice. Mix into a paste and apply directly to area. Do not use oils or hot water on the affected skin. Help it dry out, but don't get sunburned.

Puncture wounds   Let blood wash out wound. Apply pressure with a clean cloth when you want to stop bleeding. Cold water relieves pain and swelling. Keep protected from dirt by bandaging with clean cloth.

Sprains   Immobilize the weakened part. Apply cool water to bring down swelling and ease pain. Six to eight hours later, when swelling has ceased, hot, then cold water compresses will aid healing through increasing circulation. Comfrey, grated potatoes, carrots are all helpful externally.

Stings and bites   Remove the stinger or the critter itself. Plantain, clay are helpful.

PRESSURE POINTS TO RELIEVE PAIN

by Michael Blate

For some time, I have taught a process called *"G-Jo"* (pronounced ji-jhiu, which means first aid in Chinese) at local (South Florida) growth centers. The process is a crude form of acupressure whose goal is the temporary relief of numerous ailments. Faced with the problem of first defining the concepts of *Ch'i,* meridians, etc., it soon became obvious that if I was to hold the attention of even my enthusiastic New Age students, something more quickly assimilable had to be presented. And since most of them merely wanted to know what to do in times of personal need, I began substituting the word, *paramedical*—meaning "that which precedes and/or supplements PROPER medical attention"—wherever applicable.

To further simplify the process, I placed my teaching emphasis upon a handful of points (of the more than one hundred available for paramedical use), easily memorizable, which are most often effective and easily found. In effect, these paramedical pressure points are broad-acting acupuncture points that have been used for centuries in a formula fashion. In short, they are "cookbook" points that may bring TEMPORARY relief from many ailments when properly located and used. I have found the results quite satisfying.

However, in no way should the use of these points be considered an alternative to proper medical attention, either of the Western or oriental variety. Good health is obviously not as simple as pressing and massaging a few body areas. But relief from pain and various discomforts may be.

Furthermore, classical acupuncture is rather specific about the direction of massage, if fingers are selected as the stimulating instrument. Either clockwise or counterclockwise might be recommended, especially for points located upon the torso. But the paramedical pressure points are located either below the elbows or below the knees —thus, not much attention needs to be paid as to the direction of massage. I have had good results using even a back and forth stimulation, though I often massage counterclockwise to help relieve pain.

There are only two steps necessary in the paramedical massage technique: Find the point; then massage it DEEPLY with the TIP (not the ball or the pad) of the finger. Or, if more pressure is needed, I sometimes use either the knuckle or the other end of a non-retractable ballpoint pen. Finding the points is quite simple, in that they will "announce" themselves with a twinge of pain or sensitivity when deeply probed. Once located, begin the massage AS DEEPLY as the sufferer can reasonably tolerate. From my experience, it is nearly axiomatic that the pain/sensitivity at the point of massage must supersede the pain being treated. With rare exception, the pain at the pressure point will subside soon after the massage has been completed; usually immediately after.

Feedback, if the sufferer is other than oneself, is essential. Verbal is good; but when a point is located, quite often the sufferer will grimace, make a small cry, or twitch. "How does that feel?" or "Is this the point?" should be asked after telling him he will notice a distinct difference between the point and the surrounding area. Again, THE MOST PAINFUL OR SENSITIVE SPOT IS THE ONE TO MASSAGE.

AND WHILE IT IS DIFFICULT TO MASSAGE THE POINT TOO DEEPLY (within humane limits), IT IS QUITE EASY *NOT* TO MASSAGE THE POINT DEEPLY ENOUGH. When massaging the point, THE FINGER SHOULD NOT MOVE ACROSS OR AROUND THE SKIN, BUT THE MASSAGER'S FINGER AND THE SUFFERER'S SKIN SHOULD MOVE TOGETHER. It is my experience that if no relief is gotten, it is probable that either a too-shallow or gentle massage or the improper selection of the point is the fault.

Those familiar with acupuncture will recognize the following points as: LARGE INTESTINE 4; LUNG 7; STOMACH 36; BLADDER 60; SPLEEN 6; TRIPLE-WARMER 5; and PERICARDIUM (or CIRCULATION-SEX) 6. For our purposes, however, these names are unnecessary. The locations described and illustrated are APPROXIMATE; searching for the precise spot should be begun at the area described. Then work carefully, deeply, around the area until the point "announces" itself.

Under the column headed "POSSIBLE USES," the affected areas or symptoms defined do not necessarily represent the entire scope of uses each point may have, or that it is necessarily the single best point that an experienced acupuncturist might choose. Their selection is a culmination of my personal research in nearly every book (in English) on the subject, conversations with and teaching of masters of acupuncture, and—perhaps most important—my own experience with hundreds of students and sufferers.

In my experience, the rate of success is greatest in problems of non-chronic pain and least successful with ailments of a long-standing nature. Minor accidents or other onetime ailments present the ideal opportunity for their use; likewise, headaches, neuralgia, and other aches often respond well to the following points' proper massage. For our purposes, accident and disease (dis-ease, really) are considered the same. Relief may be complete—as it often is when performed by one experienced in the technique—or partial; but generally there is some. And it is felt immediately after the massage has been completed, if it has been properly done.

The massage should be begun as quickly as possible after the symptoms present themselves, and should be done bilaterally. That is, when one point (say, point number 1) is massaged on one hand, then the same point should be massaged for an equal length of time on the opposite hand.

To digress a moment, locating acupuncture points has always been a difficult task, in that a number of complex measurements of the SUFFERER'S (or patient's) body are needed to determine accurately the tiny (some say not wider than one or two centimeters) points before proper acupuncture can be done. In other words, there are only relative measurements (relative exclusively to the patient/sufferer) and numerous formulas exist. But for the purposes of the paramedical massage, only two measurements are necessary to remember: the WIDTH OF THE SUFFERER'S THUMB AT ITS WIDEST POINT (generally just behind the nail); and the WIDTH OF THE SUFFERER'S HAND, MEASURED ACROSS THE REARMOST KNUCKLES (toward the wrist), not including the thumb. (Plate I, line A)

POINT ⚹   APPROXIMATE LOCATION   POSSIBLE USES

1. In the webbing between thumb and forefinger. First, squeeze the thumb and forefinger together and find the mound in the webbing. Place one finger on the top of the mound and relax the hand. Begin probing, then massage. See Plate I.

This is the first point to think of for any problem that occurs above the neck. Problems of the face, ears, tongue, sinuses, etc., as well as those of shoulders, neck, and the respiratory system may often be temporarily relieved with this point.

2. The width of one thumb above the wrist (toward the elbow), along the top edge of the forearm, in line with the thumbnail. This is a difficult point to find as it is buried in a small hollow; but if one will join the webbing of the thumbs (Plate II) so that the index finger falls along the top of the forearm, the tip of the

As with point number 1, this point may be helpful with most problems of the head and neck. Additionally, problems of the lungs and chest may respond favorably to this point. This point, alone or in conjunction with point number 1,

PLATE I

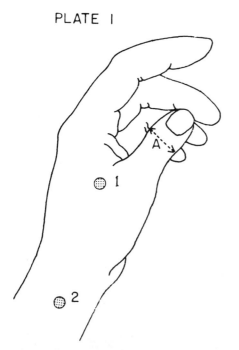

PLATE II

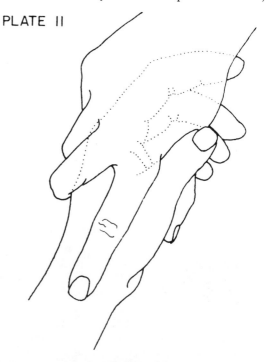

POINT ⚔   APPROXIMATE LOCATION   POSSIBLE USES

index finger (relaxed) will rest directly atop this point.   may be tried for any problem above the
See Plates I and II.   upper abdomen.

3. The width of one hand (measured across the knuckles)   One of the most "potent" paramedical
    below the bottom of the kneecap, then move slightly   points on the body. It is used with any
    to the OUTSIDE of the leg. This point will be found   problem that occurs below the chest,
    between the bone (tibia) and the muscle, in a small   and some use it in combination with any
    "trough." While it may be difficult to find at first, with   other point to treat any problem. Any
    some practice this point may be easily located and   gastric problem, especially when used
    massaged with the knuckle of the index finger. See   with point number 5, may be reduced
    Plate III.   or relieved.

4. In the valley behind the OUTER ankle, between the   This is a general pain-relief center for
    crown of the ankle and the Achilles' tendon. See   the entire body. While there may be
    Plate III.   more effective points for specific areas,
                                                                 this may be tried as a first or last
                                                                 resort. This point is also effective for
                                                                 problems of the leg, foot, back, etc.

PLATE III

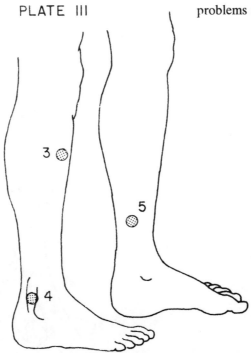

POINT ⚹   APPROXIMATE LOCATION   POSSIBLE USES

5. The width of one hand ABOVE the crown of the
    INNER ANKLE, very close, or atop the trailing edge
    of the bone (tibia). By running one's finger up the edge
    of the bone, one invariably finds a very tender spot.
    This is the point. See Plate III.

This point, especially when used in
conjunction with point number 3, may
be helpful with problems of the lower
abdomen, the sexual and reproductive
organs (including menstruation
discomfort), the legs, feet, and back,
etc.

These basic acupressure points and many others
are described and illustrated in *The Natural
Healer's Acupressure Handbook.* If you want
more information on G-Jo, write to:

The G-Jo Institute
Box 8060
Hollywood, Florida 33024

HEADACHE RELIEF

by Denni McCarthy

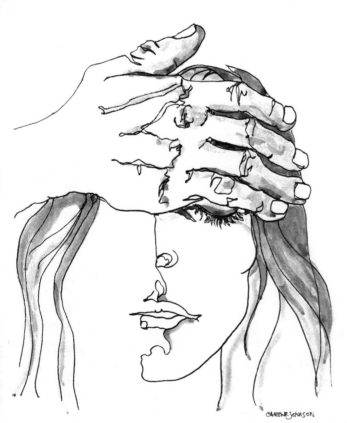

CAROLE JOHNSON

Headaches have visited me often over the last few years. I've learned a lot about how to deal with them and how to read their message. A headache is usually the body's signal that toxins have accumulated and aren't being eliminated properly. Tension and constipation (insufficient elimination or digestion) are probably present and need to be dealt with first. Your body needs to rest, relax, and get back into a harmonious balance.

FACE SAUNAS, BATHS, HERBS

One of the first things I do is prepare an herbal face sauna using spearmint, chamomile, and rosemary. I put one handful of each herb in a quart of boiled water and steep it for twenty minutes. Then I put a towel over my head and the pot, inhaling the healing steam for five to twenty minutes. This stimulates the skin and circulation, releases sweat, and helps unclog whatever is blocked. I've also used a drop of peppermint and eucalyptus oils in one quart of hot water in the same way. This "sauna" not only opened my clogged sinuses but also caused my entire body to sweat, encouraging the eliminative process. I followed this treatment with a cold rinse of pure water and felt rejuvenation beginning. If you're feeling particularly tense, a hot bath with the same herbs and oils adding some catnip, hops, or valerian root, will be very relaxing. A hot foot bath will have the same effect. I also drink a cupful of strong peppermint tea (two teaspoons per cup of hot water) adding some valerian as a nervine (½ teaspoon). If you're lucky enough to know of a large mint garden you might go and lie down in the middle of it, letting the healing essence of the herb soothe your brain.

REST, BREATHING VISUALIZATION

After bathing and drinking the herbs, I put myself in a relaxing situation, usually in bed where it is quiet and warm. Often I'll fall asleep and wake up refreshed, my headache gone. Or I might begin to do some deep breathing, bringing healing breath into each part of my body on the inhalation and sending the disease and tension out on the exhalation. This technique, along with visualizing the actual pain in my head, its exact location, size, shape, and then its leaving, can be very effective. Breath is a great relaxer and can often quiet a tense and uncomfortable mind and body.

FASTING AND MASSAGING

It's important to let your whole system have a food rest as well. It's probably already over-loaded and needs some time to complete its digestive and eliminative processes. So give yourself the treat of fasting, and drink some herbal teas or cool water. When you begin to feel better have some vegetable juice or vegetable broth. Remember, you're doing yourself a favor by not eating.

A massage is also helpful when you have a headache. The G-Jo points as discussed earlier brought me relief. You can do a self-massage or ask a friend to treat you. The feet can also be massaged; as sensitive receivers for all the organs of the body, they aid the entire system. The head reflexes are located on the underside of the toes from the base to the tip. The whole foot should be massaged with a firm pressure so that other points such as the liver, stomach, and intestines are energized. A little "tiger-balm" or other healing liniment rubbed into the temples, forehead, and back of the neck (PLEASE, NOT IN THE EYES!) is very soothing. All these various reflex points and direct massage aid the body as it begins to heal itself, and provide a means for sending energy to the diseased areas.

These are some of the ways I've learned to work with headaches to heal myself. It's also important to become sensitive to preventing them. Awareness of diet, exercise, relaxation, etc., is the first step to a healthy body. There is no one cure for a headache, but there are many natural ways to deal with it and many ways you can help yourself to prevent its repeated occurrence.

AT LAST!
A "CURE FOR THE COMMON COLD"

From the laboratory of common experience and the text of old herbals comes modern science's impossible dream: a cure for the common cold. Fortunately you don't have to just take a pill that dries your symptoms up. This treatment involves *you* in the process of alleviating the underlying cause—CONGESTION. Long before congestion appears as mucus escaping through a runny nose, the body has begun backing up in the digestive system and the pores. By opening the skin's pores and by stimulating normal bowel elimination, *you* can dramatically stop an early-stage cold.

Usually the first early warnings of a common cold are an achy head, stuffiness, and aches and pains in other body parts. Think about how a cold comes on for you. Set your mind now to notice those early warnings and find time for this treatment.

The symptoms of a cold may be the early stages of other diseases such as mumps, measles, bronchial problems, etc. If these conditions develop, treat them accordingly. If symptoms persist and you seem to be getting nowhere with the treatment you are using, see a competent wholistic physician.

INITIALLY

1. Draw a hot, steamy bath.
2. Make a four-cup pot of tea, equal parts yarrow, elder flower, hyssop, and peppermint.
3. Put it by your bedside to steep—strainer and anything else needed too.
4. Drink one glass distilled water with up to ½ teaspoon salt dissolved in it.
5. Get in your *hot* bath for fifteen minutes. Add a few drops of eucalyptus oil if you wish . . . it helps the head and chest open up.
6. Towel off quickly.
7. Jump into a very warm bed—lots of blankets.
8. Start drinking your herb tea and drink a cup every half hour until you get a good sweat going.
9. Stay in bed for a while or overnight—be sure you have stopped sweating and feel rested.
10. Sponge off with warm water with a little vinegar in it to disinfect your pores.

11. Be happy, don't worry about your vinegary smell, and don't try to do too much work for a day or so.

12. If there are no further complications, follow up with an ongoing tea of peppermint, lemon, garlic, and honey.

IF'S

If you want to completely escape the symptoms of a cold, you must notice the early warnings and act within six to twelve hours.

If you are already experiencing a cold, flu, or fever, the treatment will certainly make you feel better but not necessarily completely alleviate the symptoms.

If your symptoms are stronger than normal or if you feel constipated, add an enema before the bath.

If you feel quite weak, add a salt glow after the bath. See *Bath to Eden* by Jethro Kloss for instructions.

If your child seems to need this treatment go ahead if the child is older. For younger children or babies use a different treatment. First rub oil and then pressed garlic all over the soles of their feet. Then put on warm socks and bundle them up under lots of blankets. This will open their pores, cause sweating, and break up obstructions in their bodies. Keep them bundled up until their body temperature is normal and they are feeling better. Then sponge them off with warm water with a little vinegar in it. Keep the child warm during this process. Do a light massage (meridians if you know them) to finish up. You'll be able to notice an interesting effect of the garlic. It will travel all the way through your child's body and you'll begin to smell it on the child's breath after very few minutes.

FINAL THOUGHTS

Here are a few counterindications. If you have any of these conditions, don't use this treatment: fever due to concussion; low blood pressure; poison ivy, sumac, or oak; a pain in the abdomen near the appendix.

Go easy on your food intake till you are well past the symptoms.

Remember, you are assisting nature in curing the common cold. You are not really the curer. The body simply wants to heal itself and regain balance. The commonest ailments will respond to natural treatments when we understand what our bodies want to do to achieve that balance.

SOME SUMMER SUGGESTIONS

by Rosemary Gladstar

Since ancient days, like a ritual, we welcome the warmth and aroma of summer. It comes, a jovial friend willing to take us anywhere in its sun-bronzed arms.

But like each season it too has its woes. The sun whose rays we bask beneath can burn as painfully as fire; the warmth that beckons the flowers to bloom arouses dormant poison oak and gives birth to mosquitoes, fleas, and flies.

Nature provides her remedies in season. It takes only a small amount of time to prepare these protective aids.

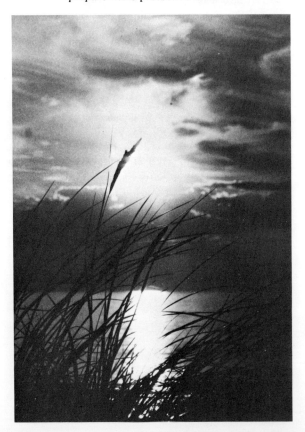

SUNBURN

A good protective oil is made of:

½ cup olive oil
2 tablespoons apple cider vinegar
2 tablespoons rose water or orange flower water
50,000 units vitamin E oil
Shake well before using.

Another soothing lotion is made by soaking thin cucumber slices in buttermilk or yoghurt. Use the cucumber as a pad to apply this wonderful skin tonic to burned areas. Cucumbers aid in lowering body temperature and are great summer coolers. My grandmother always had cooling salads of cucumber, garlic, and yoghurt in the summer. When we were hot, she served us this creamy goodness; and when we burned, she patted this tonic on our burning bodies.

Mix equal amounts aloe vera gel, apple cider vinegar, and vitamin E oil for another super burn salve.

If you do get a burn, shower immediately with *cold* water. (Your skin will continue to burn unless you quench that flame.) Mix equal amounts apple cider vinegar and rose water and apply with cotton pads to entire burned area.

For peeling skin, brew a strong tea of papaya leaf, two tablespoons herb to one cup water, strain and apply. Do not wipe off. Or better, mash a ripe papaya and apply to peeling area. Papaya aids in removing dead cells while toning the skin.

PESTS

Insect-repellent oils often prove invaluable in the early evenings of summer. Pennyroyal, eucalyptus, citronella, and rosemary are oils famed for their insect-repellent properties. Use either alone or in combinations. Pennyroyal is the most effective. Dab the oil on clothing or on areas where protection is needed. If you wish to rub directly on skin, dilute the insect-repellent oils with a small amount of apricot or almond oil.

Pets suffer needlessly from fleas in the spring and fall. Wash your pet once a week for three consecutive weeks with a strong solution of pennyroyal tea. This will remove the eggs. After washing, *lightly* rub pennyroyal oil over animals' fur. (They do not like the smell at first.) You should also make a flea collar: soak a leather strip or heavy cord in pennyroyal oil twenty-four hours and tie around pet's neck.

In France pots of basil are placed on tables to repel flies. Fresh sprigs of bay leaves do the same. What more pleasant way to protect one's house than basil growing about, bay tucked in the corners, and fennel over the door.

DRY SKIN AND HAIR

I love to play with God; ocean waves to dance with, wind to sing about, golden sun rays engulf like a warming lover. But hair and skin become parched by overexposure to summer elements. Anoint your hair with rosemary oil. A tiny drop rubbed on the ends of your hair will condition, strengthen, and protect it. If you're to be in the sun for a long time, oil your hair slightly more than usual and loosely braid for extra protection.

Sun hats are great! They protect your face, your hair, and really add to the costume. I bought mine on special at the Guerneville five-and-ten; decorated it with ribbons and flowers from the field. It looks and smells divine.

For dry skin, create a protective oil. Use in bath or massage into skin. ¼ cup apricot oil, ¼ cup almond oil, ¼ cup avocado oil, 100,000 units vitamin A, 50,000 units vitamin E. Mix together and store in closed container. Scent with a favorite essential oil. Sesame seed and olive oil (strong scent) are also wonderful oils for your skin.

POISON OAK

A small book could be written on oak remedies; out of frustration so many things have been tried. Drink witch hazel bark or white oak bark tea, ¼ cup three times a day every day until poison oak is gone. A powerful liniment consists of one ounce goldenseal powder, one ounce myrrh gum powder, ½ ounce cayenne, and ½ ounce grindelia. Steep in two pints alcohol seven days. Strain and bottle for use. Apply every ½ hour to poison oak. *Be consistent.* Fels-Naptha is an old-fashioned bar soap very useful in washing poison oak oil from your skin when you first come in contact.

Salt and vinegar rubbed on is another patent remedy. Very strong, however; if your skin's sensitive, dilute with a little rose water.

Out in the field, mountains, far from home and

you start to itch with poison oak, gather plantain, dock, or chickweed. Mash and apply the fresh juice over rash. Horsetail herb is another of nature's cures. Simmer ¼ cup horsetail in one cup cider vinegar twenty minutes. Strain and store in refrigerator. Just before you apply, dilute with buttermilk or yoghurt. Do not scratch poison oak and do not use an oil remedy. Be consistent, apply remedy every ½ hour.

(EDITOR'S NOTE: *Our favorite poison oak remedy is mugwort tea. Use cold to wash the body, it will remove oils from the skin surface, thereby removing the irritant.*)

SUMMER COOLERS

Iced tea is among the most refreshing drinks of summer. Unlike milkshakes, thick or sweet drinks, tea actually quenches thirst.

My favorite mixture: ½ ounce hibiscus, ½ ounce lemon grass, ½ ounce strawberry leaf, ½ ounce peppermint, ½ ounce orange peel, ½ ounce cinnamon bark. Toss a handful into a gallon jug and set in the sunshine in the afternoon. Refrigerate that night and it's ready. Cool and refreshing the next day. If you wish to sweeten, warm a little honey, slice an orange, and add to the jug.

Both strawberry and raspberry leaf reduce body temperature and make refreshing summer drinks. Cucumber juice is a real cooler!

Make a strong peppermint/cinnamon bark tea, sweeten with honey, and add apple juice to taste. Freeze for a treat for all.

You all should cultivate a patch of mint in your garden. In the heat of the day, gather a handful fresh. Blend with ice cubes and orange juice—delicious! Without the orange juice it is a great skin toner.

When traveling, go well stocked with jugs of iced tea. (Make it strong to allow for ice melt-age.) Take along a special jug of iced strawberry leaf tea to wash with when the sweat starts rolling. Place towels of this cooling mixture on soles of feet.

Keep cool and comfortable, enjoy the summer days while they're here.

POISON OAK, IVY, AND SUMAC:
Nature's Itch and How to Treat It

by William LeSassier

During the course of history many vegetable substances were noticed as causing irritation. These were classified under the term dermatitis venenata. Some of the many substances which can cause allergic reaction are: arnica, mustard, rue, brewer's yeast, capsicum, cantharides, mercury, turpentine, iodine, nettle, dye stuffs, primrose, cowhage, balm of Gilead, nasturtium, smartweed, podophyllum (American mandrake), oleander, and especially poison oak, sumac, and ivy. The active principle in these last four is an acid—toxicodendric acid.

People have noticed that immunity to poison oak or ivy can be a random thing, and that a person can outgrow one's immunity.

The usual process in getting poison oak or ivy is contact with the plant by touch, breathing the vapor or pollens, or breathing poison oak or ivy smoke. (This has been known to cause death.) The most active time of the year for poison oak or ivy is when it is pollenating (late May in California). The roots are most potent in winter months, leaves when they turn shiny in late spring, and berries in late summer. All parts of the plant are toxic. Once the hands contact the plant the oils are easily spread to more sensitive skin on the body: genitals, stomach area, nasal membrane, etc. Then this is carried by the blood stream into many parts of the body.

Treatment of poison oak, etc., can be done internally and externally.

EXTERNAL TREATMENT

Poultices made of chlorophyll (alkaline) plants:

mugwort
baccharius (coyote bush)
plantain
California bee plant
malva greens

To make a poultice simply crush the plants between two hard substances. Apply to the affected area. Use whatever is on hand; almost any high chlorophyll substance will work. People have used celery juice externally and internally with great success.

For total body exposure, an alkaline bath of one pound baking soda and one pound sea salt can be helpful. Also 2 pounds fresh mugwort simmered in 1½ quarts water, strained, and added to a tubful of water are useful. Both of the above baths are *alkaline* and should be taken lukewarm (about body temperature).

INTERNAL TREATMENT

The diet should be alkaline as much as possible. This would include most green foods. The sulphur vegetables (watercress, cauliflower, nasturtium, Brussels sprouts, cabbage) should be omitted. The sulphur activity might be irritating to the skin. Citrus fruits should also be omitted from the diet because of their irritating effect on the skin. Diet can include most other fruits, sprouts, seeds, etc. A very good combination of juices is parsley, celery, and romaine lettuce taken internally (three four-ounce servings daily). This seems to aid also the accompanying edema (swelling in tissues) that can be present in a person who has poison oak, ivy, or sumac by aiding moisture elimination through the kidneys. Vitamin B is excellent.

Also, homeopathic medicine offers excellent remedies for poison oak, ivy, and sumac. These, of course, vary according to the individual temperament of the patient. Consult your local homeopath for both prevention and cure of allergic reactions of poison oak, ivy, and sumac.

PREVENTION

A very good preventive is to rub fresh mugwort over the body before going out. Remedies such as "Immun Oak," a homeopathic preparation, are safe and effective. Also, eating romaine lettuce seems to help build resistance. Immediately after exposure, wash off with mugwort tea (prepare it in advance if you think you'll be exposed). Mugwort removes the surface oils from the skin. Heat opens the pores, driving the oils in, so make sure the tea is cool before using it.

The Indians used special teas made of the roots of poison oak or ivy collected in the dormant seasons. (The recipe is purposely omitted.) I do not suggest you go out and try this. They often ate the young green leaves.

While on an herb walk in California I saw a person quickly snatch a poison oak leaf and begin to munch it. He explained that he had once been afflicted by poison oak but ever since eating a few leaves every spring he was no longer bothered by it. I do not necessarily recommend this but it could be a possibility.

There are some far-reaching reasons for poison oak and ivy reactions, such as lack of attunement to the environment, allergic adrenal responses, or excessive fear. Weak skin that is overly sensitive to sunlight could also be the cause. I personally think poison oak, ivy, and sumac are protective plants, important members of the woodland community. Certainly these plants have caused many people to watch their step when hiking, as opposed to the usual trampling effect of most people. I do not mean this to be negative to people who get poison oak.

I would suggest greater etheric attunement in general by eating local plants. Find people who can identity the plants in your area. These plants are rich sources of minerals and vitamins. On the vibrational level they also provide attunement to the environment as it changes with the seasons.

A True Life Poison Oak Adventure

I recently had a good case of poison oak and was able to try out some of the typical remedies. I had been out in the country digging *ceanothus* roots, and although no poison oak leaves were visible, I apparently dug into some poison oak roots. By the following afternoon, I noticed vague irritation around my eyes and face. I made mugwort tea, let it cool, and applied it two or three times before going to bed. In the night I began to feel my face swell, and by morning I had a fat, hot, red face—my eyes swollen half shut. I normally wash off with mugwort tea immediately after exposure, and this always works. But I guess this time it was too late. I had it!

This called for definite action. First Barbara blended up a poultice of plantain and that helped some. Next we tried a poultice of celery, vinegar, and a little tofu added to make a paste. I could really feel the difference after the celery. The swelling reduced slightly and it felt less irritated.

Meanwhile, my stomach and hands started breaking out but not swelling like my face. I tried mugwort tea, goldenseal, and vinegar, and then Christine suggested the inner gel of aloe vera. The aloe worked the best, drawing, drying, and stopping the itching pretty effectively.

Barbara lit some frankincense and myrrh, and put some soothing music and another celery poultice on. I forgot about work and started reading the *Narnia* books by C. S. Lewis. But we weren't done yet. Next we tried a paste of ground oatmeal. It took a long time to dry (never did completely) and boy, did we have a time trying to get it all off my face, chest, stomach, legs, and hands. It was like a gooey glue. If I had taken the bath William suggests, I'm sure it would have come off easier. In any case, it didn't work as well as the aloe vera on the rash and the celery paste on the swelling. Oh, well, another true life adventure.   D.C.

YOGA FOR AN ACHING BACK

by Larry and Sandy Shaw

Surveys conducted by the National Center for Health indicate that almost eight million Americans are being treated for chronic back pain, and two million new cases are added each year. Back pain is one of the most common complaints of our modern life, and as our life-style becomes more hectic this figure can only increase. Diagnosing the cause of back problems is very difficult. Many backaches are caused by displaced or malfunctioning organs, such as kidneys, bladder, and prostate. Stomach ailments can also manifest as lower back pain. But far and away the major cause of "the Great American Backache" is disorders of the spine and inordinately weak back muscles.

Our sedentary life-styles are primarily responsible for the muscular weakness in the back. Body fat (almost all of us carry too much weight), poor posture (take a look at your own and the posture of those around you), lack of proper exercise (not just a once-a-week tennis game or jog around the block), tension and stress (manifest as muscular tension) are other contributing causes. The design of our modern furniture and automobile seats only adds to the scope of the problem.

Since Hatha Yoga postures are both preventive and curative, the following exercises can be used to relieve pain if you are already suffering; or to tone, strengthen, and stretch the back muscles as an ounce of prevention. You can practice Hatha Yoga just about anywhere, inside or outside. Pick a clean place that is flat and practice on a blanket or mat. In the beginning pick a quiet place so that you will not be distracted. As the concentration improves, the mind won't so easily wander. Practice the Hatha Yoga exercises (called postures) slowly and deliberately. Hold each posture as long as you can without undue strain or pain to any part of the body. Don't move about, hold very still. Mentally release the tension barriers and *relax* into the posture. Always rest between the postures so that you can rejuvenate before starting the next posture.

SPINAL ROCK

The rocking motion of the Spinal Rock eases tension in the back and shoulders, and massages the back muscles. The spine and nerve trunks are also stimulated. Warm up with the Spinal Rock before attempting any of the other Hatha Yoga postures. The Spinal Rock warms the body and gives energy. (EDITOR'S NOTE: *For these rocking and rolling postures, we re-emphasize using a folded blanket or mat to protect your vertebrae from the hard floor. Better yet, do your postures on a nice, soft, green lawn . . . nature's Yoga mat.)*

1. Sit on the floor. Bend your knees, sliding your heels toward the buttocks, and grasp your legs, just above the knee joints. Drop your head forward.

2. INHALE, and gently rock/roll back over your spine and back muscles. Stretch the legs over your head as far as you can, without straining. At first, keep your knees slightly bent.

3. EXHALE, and rock back and forward over your spine to the original sitting position.

4. Continue to rock back and forth over your spine and back as *slowly* as possible. Rock until you grow tired, then lie flat on your back and rest. Breathe deeply, through the nose, and keep the breath very slow and smooth.

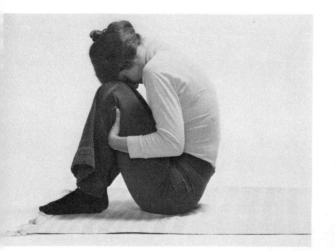
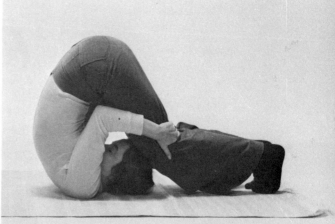
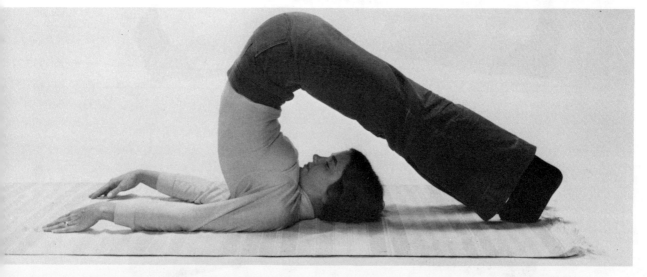

TORTOISE VARIATION

The Tortoise Variation tones the sciatic nerve and muscles of the lower back, relieving the pain of sciatica and lumbago. This posture is designed for maximum flexibility of the hamstrings, as well as the lumbar region and the ligaments. Each side of the lower back receives an extended stretch.

1. Sit on the floor, with the legs stretched wide. Reach arms up over your head, then, bending, reach down toward the *right* leg. Hold onto the leg, ankle, or foot.

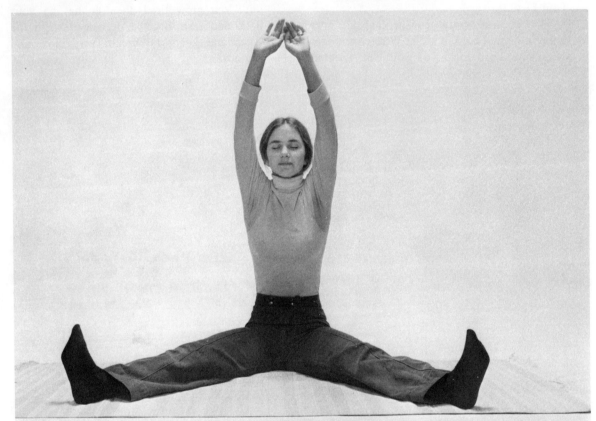

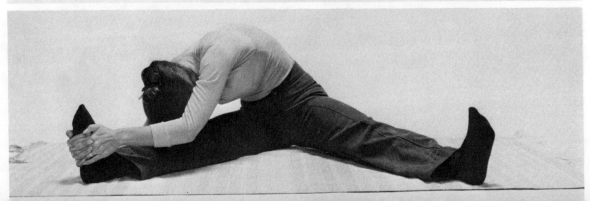

2. Don't strain. Attempt to relax the muscles. Mentally monitor your body. Breathe normally. Hold position as long as you can without strain. Then relax.
3. Reach arms up over head again, then bend and reach for *left* leg, repeating exercise.
4. Lie flat on your back and rest. Breathe deeply before continuing with the next posture.

CAMEL

The Camel tones and strengthens the muscles of the spine and gives it greater elasticity. This posture will also correct any displacements in the vertebrae and will strengthen the neck and shoulders. Those who suffer from hunched back should practice this posture, since the whole spine is stretched backward and toned.

1. Kneel on the floor, knees about six inches apart. Bend head and neck backward, curving the spine backward as well, and push the pelvic area forward.
2. Lower your hands to your heels (you may not be able to reach them on first try) and support body by resting your feet. Don't strain, but hold as long as you comfortably can. Breathe deeply. Concentrate on relaxing your back muscles.
3. Release slowly by straightening back up. Lie on your back and rest, breathing deeply.

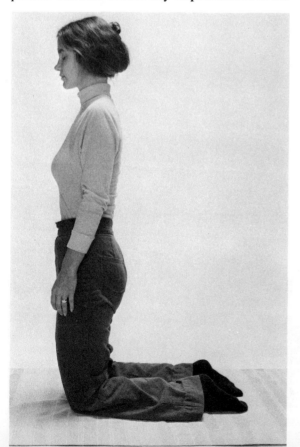

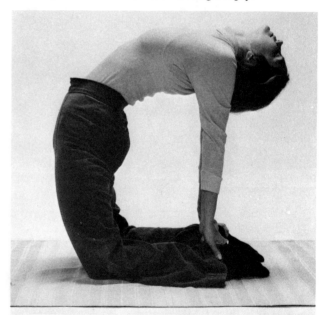

PLOUGH

Spinal flexibility is a major benefit of the Plough. Due to the forward bend, the spine receives an extra supply of blood, nourishing the spine and nerve trunks. This posture is of great help to those suffering backaches and arthritis of the back. The Plough rejuvenates the sex glands, liver, kidneys, and the spleen. The neck is also strengthened, and the thyroid stimulated, thus helping regulate the weight.

1. Sit on the floor and bend your knees, sliding your heels toward the buttocks. Drop your head forward.
2. *Slowly* rock/roll back over your spine and back muscles. Stretch the legs over the head as far as you can without straining. Lower hands to the floor, palms down (you may not be able to place your toes on the floor at first). Don't strain. Relax the whole body and focus your attention into the body. Breathe normally. Hold as long as you can without straining.
3. Bend knees to the forehead, place your hands behind the knees and rock forward. Rest, lying on your back, while breathing deeply.

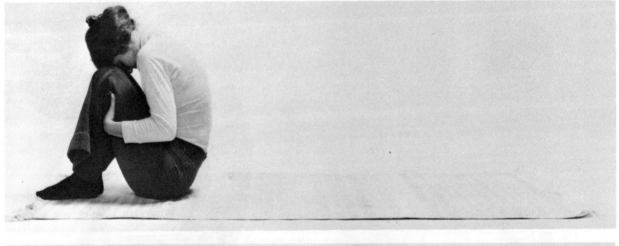

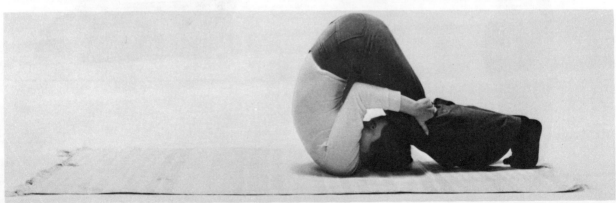

COBRA

In the Cobra posture the deep and superficial muscles of the back are well toned. The spinal region is toned, and those suffering from slight displacements of spinal discs can use the Cobra to replace the discs in their original positions. All the vertebrae and their ligaments are pulled backward and receive a rich supply of blood. The internal abdominal organs are toned and the abdominal muscles are pulled and strengthened.

1.   Lie on the floor, face down. Rest the palms of the hands on the floor near your shoulders, elbows up and in.

2.   Raise forehead from the floor, and extend your chin. *Slowly,* pushing down with hands, lift your chest from the floor. Attempt to straighten the elbows, keeping shoulders relaxed. Flex the buttocks and stretch the front of your body.

3.   Breathe normally. Hold the position until you grow tired.

4.   *Slowly* lower down, and touch your forehead to the floor. Release your arms. Relax, lying on your stomach, and breathe deep, slow breaths.

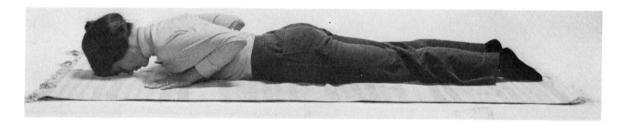

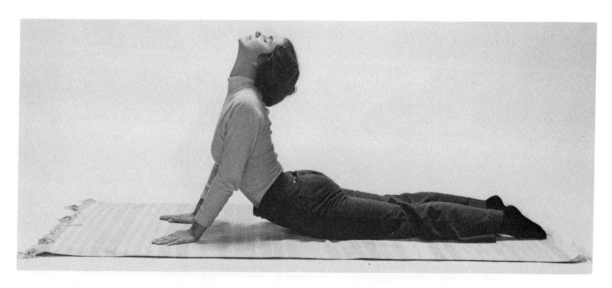

BOW

The Bow brings elasticity to the spine and massages the back muscles. Persons suffering from disc problems may find relief by the regular practice of this posture. The abdominal muscles are toned and this posture removes constipation and helps to cure dyspepsia, rheumatism, and gastrointestinal disorders. It also reduces fat, aids digestion, and invigorates the appetite.

1. Lie on your stomach and bend your knees. Reach back with the hands and hold onto your ankles. Lift the chest and thighs from the floor, arching your body backwards. Only the abdomen bears the weight of the body.

2. Hold as long as you can without straining. Hold the mind still and focus on the body. Breathe evenly.

3. *Slowly* lower down, release the arms, and rest on the stomach. Breathe deeply.

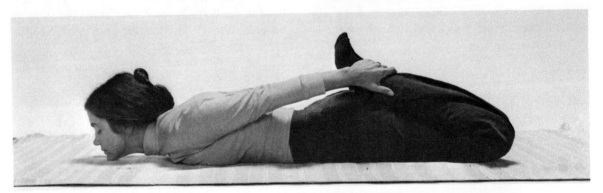

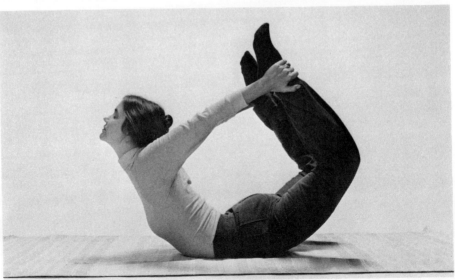

EASY TWIST

If you have a lower backache, practice this position. The spine must bend in six different directions for maximum flexibility and health; forward and backward, from side to side, as well as twisting laterally. The Easy Twist provides a corkscrew twisting motion for the spine, which keeps it elastic and relaxed. The spinal nerve roots and the sympathetic system are toned, calming the nervous system. With this posture, the back muscles are massaged and tension released from the shoulders. The kidneys, spleen, liver, and abdominal organs are also toned.

1.   Lie on your back. Stretch your arms out from the shoulders, forming a "T" with your body. Bend your knees and lift them toward your chest.

2.   Lower your knees to the floor, sideways to the right, turning your head in the opposite direction. Keep your shoulders flat on the floor.

3.   Hold in this twist as long as you comfortably can. Breathe normally.

4.   Twist back to the original position and repeat posture on opposite side.

5.   After completing the posture, rest on your back and breathe deep, slow breaths.

Larry and Sandy Shaw have taught yoga for over five years in the San Diego area. Their book, *Yoga Warm-ups for Joggers, Runners and Bicyclers,* will be published soon by Bookmakers. They are beginning a yoga retreat center in Fayetteville, Arkansas.

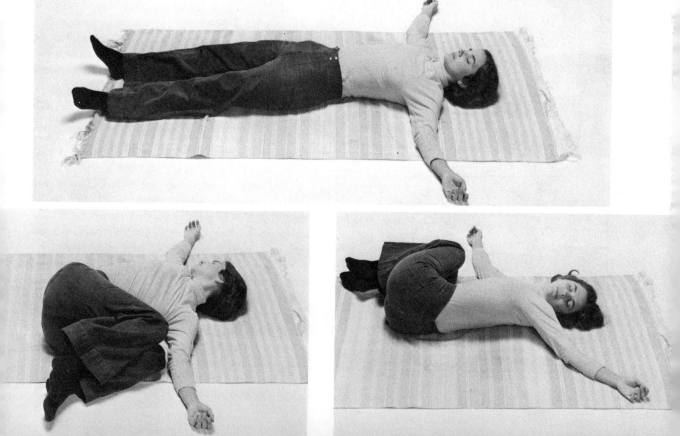

HEPATITIS:
Meeting the Liver the Hard Way

by Allan Jaklich

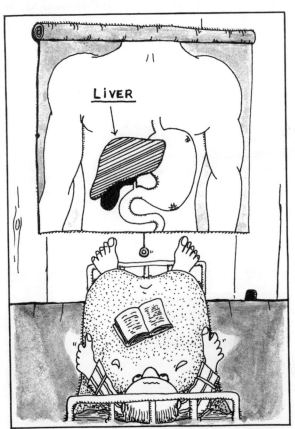

Three springs ago I limped back home after a grueling, three-month trip "south of the border." The journey had been plagued with tropical maladies, such as dysentery and staph. Already exhausted, I capped my trip with a marathon ride home—from Huehuetenango, Guatemala, to California—in a VW bus cramped with blankets, baskets, four people, and a German shepherd dog.

One of my traveling companions, it turned out, had been exposed to and was coming down with hepatitis. Just a few days later, after I returned to the sleepy mountain community I called home, "hep" knocked me flat on my back.

The initial attack was the worst. I was too weak to move from bed, and too nauseous to eat anything. The first few nights' sleep were difficult. I was achy, shaky, feverish, and wet with perspiration. All the symptoms of hep manifested: my urine turned brown, my feces lost their normal dark color, and worst of all, my body turned a sickly yellow!

The intense attack lasted a few days, during which time all I could do was suffer and let hep take its course. The two friends I shared a house with, and the four others living on our homestead, brought smiles, teas, and broths. Within four days, I recovered enough strength to begin poring through the small library of self-healing books that I could, literally, reach from my bed! (One of the interests that drew our community together was natural healing.)

In *Healing Yourself,* I found that there are two common types of Hep. (1) "Infectious Hepatitis," is a virus passed from person to person orally through the mucous membranes (like partaking from the same glass, or from a sneeze). This is the most common hep, and the one I experienced. (2) "Serum Hepatitis" is more severe, and is usually transmitted through hypodermic needles. Hep can be caused by toxins as well.

I assumed "infectious" meant anyone I came in contact with would "catch" hep. So to protect my companions, I kept one set of dishes aside for myself, and washed them separately in very hot water. Friends brought herbs and fresh honey from our hives, but kept their distance. "We" tried to keep "them" from touching "my" mucus . . . in as comfortable a way as possible. And no one seemed overly concerned that I might be a "carrier," which contributed greatly to the healing atmosphere.

It turns out that "infectious" does not mean "contagious." I'm thankful that not one of the sixteen people I came in contact with during my hep "caught" it. So don't panic, even if you are exposed to hep. Some people are susceptible to infectious hepatitis, and others aren't, depending on their health (I was an exhausted and ripe candidate).

THE LIVER

Hepatitis is a disease or inflammation of the liver. Raymond Dextreit, in his book, *Our Earth Our Cure,* devotes thirty pages to this "unknown

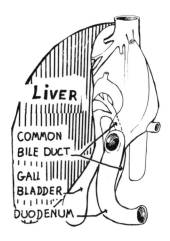

organ." The liver was indeed unknown to me (my tropical diseases made me aware just how little I knew about my organs). But when I pushed my fingers up under my right rib cage, there it was—and tender to the touch—my liver.

The liver is our largest organ, and so important, according to Dextreit, that if it is not healthy, the body cannot be well. It will take a lot of abuse before showing symptoms (the liver can be 80 per cent non-functioning and still serve the body admirably). But once pushed beyond its capacities, recovery is slow.

The liver is a main organ of digestion. It secretes about a quart of bile (digestive juice) into the intestines each day. (Bile predigests fats, lubricates and stimulates the digestive process, regulates intestinal flora, and helps keep worms in check.) But when hep attacks liver cells, bile leaks into the blood stream, causing the yellowing of skin and whites of the eyes characteristic of jaundice. With less bile in the intestines, digestion fails.

The liver forms the protein needed to replace damaged cells . . . even its own. It also stores up glycogen (for future energy needs) and vitamins

A, B₁, D, E, and K (the antihemorrhagic vitamin). What's more, the liver neutralizes poisons in the body, produces blood clotting and anticoagulant substances, regulates blood volume, and is a source of body heat and metabolic balance. That's why an ailing liver puts the body in such a tailspin!

LIVER NO-NO'S

Treating a "bad" liver requires *rest,* but this means more than simply lying around. Since digestion is impaired, overeating is to be avoided . . . as well as overcooked, refined, processed, or any other hard-to-digest foods. Fried foods are especially hard on the liver.

Chemicals, drugs, and medications—alcohol, caffeine, cocaine, nicotine, theobromine, etc.—are no-no's too, as they make the liver work extra hard to detoxify them. All are to be avoided, including coffee, black tea, and cocoa.

I recall that cottage cheese, lettuce, tomato, onion, brewer's yeast, butter, whole-wheat-bread sandwiches were very delicious "medicine."

When, during the first few weeks of hep, I was still too weak to leave bed, I continued reading about and trying various liver/hepatitis treatments.

FOODS

While hard-to-digest foods like meat are to be avoided, protein *is* needed in rebuilding the liver cells. As my appetite slowly returned, I discovered a number of vegetables—raw or lightly steamed—that provided easy-to-digest protein: sprouts, broccoli, comfrey, peas, and spinach among them.

As I felt able to handle more protein, I included yoghurt, buttermilk, kefir (three "cultured" dairy products that actually aid digestion and contribute to the balance of intestinal flora),

and soft cottage cheese to my diet, but continued to avoid the other processed, harder-to-digest dairy foods.

Every few days I'd have a poached egg (not fried) on toast, with plenty of brewer's yeast, which seemed like real "solid" food. Occasionally I'd eat almonds, Brazil nuts, walnuts, and peanuts—chewing them thoroughly for ease of digestion. Sunflower and sesame seeds were another source of protein, and brought variety to my "recovery" diet.

Some other delicious foods act as a tonic for the liver. So I happily ate cabbage, dandelion greens, garlic, and onion for their toning and cleansing effect. I often started the day with a "liver flush"—two or more garlic cloves pressed into the juice of a lemon, then mixed with a teaspoon of olive oil (it makes a great salad dressing too).

It turns out that the aromatic, powerfully fragrant herbs are those most beneficial to the liver. This includes many culinary herbs, such as rosemary and thyme. Teas of these herbs definitely have a medicinal or purifying quality about them. Mugwort grew right outside my door, so I often harvested leaves and made a tea, which acts as a nervine. Comfrey grew nearby too, and I used it in tea and salads. I also used goldenseal (also known as jaundice root), but sparingly, as it is a very powerful tonic . . . one teaspoon in a glass of water can match castor oil as a bitter medicine any day! A dose once or twice a week was plenty for me.

I tried to manage my diet so that I'd get my needed vitamins in their fresh-food form (but just in case, I also took a daily dose of vitamin "pills" . . . derived from foods). Some foods became regulars at my meals: brewer's yeast (B), kale (A), peppers (C), eggs (D), whole cereals like millet (E), and alfalfa sprouts (K).

PATIENCE

The mind must rest, as well as the liver. A friend told me that in Chinese folklore, the liver is the emotional center or the "organ of patience." So it seems that a sick liver is the sign of impatience, characterized by the harmful emotions of anger, resentment, fear, despair, etc. Patience *is* called for. An anxious mind will only prolong the malaise. (As my homestead friends went out each day to their spring garden planting chores, I had to do my own "interior chores"— letting go of feeling guilty or sorry for myself, and putting my mind at rest. So don't discount positive thought. Visualize yourself as healthy every day, and you will be . . . in time.

EXERCISE

Rest does not mean sloth. Passivity is considered as harmful to the recovering liver as fatigue, so both extremes are to be avoided. As soon as I had the strength to get up and about, I tried to get some sun and exercise each day . . . but I had to keep alert so as not to fatigue myself and cause a setback.

I got into the habit of going to a nearby meadow every morning, where the rising sun first shone into our valley. There I would begin the day with a meditation, facing the sunlight (I simply sat still and "watched" my breath). I followed that up with a regular series of exercises.

A book on Do-In I had happened to find showed self-massage techniques and acupressure points for stimulating the liver. In fact I did a series of exercises and pressure points aimed at stimulating energy flow throughout my body. So each day began with positive thought *and* action.

I usually did a few Yoga postures as well, such as the Plough (see page 110) to massage my in-

nards. Another massage for the digestion involved lying on my back and applying fingertip pressure to my organs, following a circular path from the sternum, around the navel, over the intestines, and reaching under the ribs to the sore liver.

Slowly, as my strength returned, I took on more exercise challenges: going for walks in the woods, or "down the road" to the mailbox. It was a happy day when, after a month or two, I could actually do some digging in the garden . . . if only for fifteen minutes at first.

LIFE-STYLE

During the course of my hep, some folks said, "Once you get it, you never get rid of it." That's a heavy image to lay on anyone, and I refused to accept the notion . . . believing it's possible to heal anything . . . with intelligence and faith.

But in a way they were right. The damaged liver is so slow to recover. Even *if* you do everything right, which means changing the life-style for most of us, complete healing can take up to two years. (Patience!) Now, more than three years after hep hit, a taste of alcohol, working day and night, or a few cups of coffee can still bring on exhaustion. So I still have to "watch" my liver.

Some six months after I first came down with hep, I visited an acupuncturist for a series of six needle and moxabustion (mugwort) treatments. His pulse diagnosis revealed a low-energy but improving liver, plus a few associated out-of-balance organs. The treatments definitely had a positive, balancing effect.

The best advice he gave me was to try, no matter how hard it was, to do some fasting, to give my liver a rest and chance to rebuild (he also advised that smoking marijuana—"as much as I hate to admit it"—somehow weakens the liver). It was hard, but a few three-day fasts really made an improvement in my energy. Then a year after hep, under heavy emotional circumstances, the jaundice symptoms started to return. A seven-day fast on fruit juices and vegetable broths turned it around and had me feeling more healthy than ever since the original hep attack.

FOOD FOR THE LIVER

HARD ON THE LIVER

VEGETABLES	VITAMINS	TONICS AND CLEANSERS	MENTAL ATTITUDE	HARD-TO-DIGEST FOODS
Alfalfa (and other sprouted seeds)	A—Chard, kale lamb's quarters parsley	Garlic }Lemon } "Liver Olive } Flush" Oil }	Meditation/ prayer Patience	Any processed food Beans
Broccoli	B—Bananas,	Artichoke leaves		Chocolate
Celery	bran syrup,	Beets	AROMATIC HERBS	Cocoa
Comfrey	peanuts, rice,	Carrots	Agrimony	Fried food
Dandelion	yeast	Dandelion	Blue flag*	Hard cheese
Lamb's quarters	C—Rose hips,	Honey	Centaury	Meat
Oatmeal	peppers,	Onion	Chamomile	Milk
Lima beans	mustard leaves		Clove	
Miso	D—Egg yolk,		Chicory	MEDICATIONS
Peas	milk fat	BODY THERAPY	Fennel	Alcohol
Potatoes	E—Avocado,	Acupressure	Goldenseal*	Caffeine
Millet	molasses,	Breath	Lilac	Cocaine
Rice	soybeans, whole	Do-In self-	Marigold	Marijuana
Sea weeds	cereals	massage	Mugwort	Nicotine
Spinach	K—(Antihemor-	Fasting	Nutmeg	
Watercress	rhagic) Alfalfa,	Organ massage	Pennyroyal*	BAD HABITS
Whole-wheat bread	oats, rye	Swim and sun Walks	Fumitory Rosemary	Fatigue Negative
		Work	Shepherd's purse	emotions
FRUIT	OTHER PROTEIN	Yoga postures	Tarragon	Overcooking
Apples	Brewer's yeast		Thyme	Overeating
Berries	Cottage cheese		Wild soapwort	
Grapes	Egg (poached or	CULTURED DAIRY	Woodruff	
Papaya	boiled)	Buttermilk		
	Nuts and seeds	Kefir	* Potent herbs—	
	(well chewed)	Yoghurt	use in moderation	

EPILOGUE

So my liver treatment continues, slowly becoming part of my life-style: the "liver flush," positive thought, balancing exercise with rest, pure water, raw foods, etc. Currently I'm dabbling with the curative powers of clay.

Needless to say, my advice to you is to practice preventive medicine for your liver, and abuse it as little as possible. But if you do get hep, don't panic. That just may be the opposite of patience. And there is much to learn . . . even from hepatitis.

(For those recently exposed to hepatitis, but not yet showing symptoms, M.D.s often recommend a gamma globulin shot—made up of the body's own blood protein, which has the ability to resist disease. The shot supposedly will not prevent hep, but will reduce the severity of the symptoms.)

BIBLIOGRAPHY

De Langre, Jacques. *Book of Do-In*. Japan Publications, 1977.

Dextreit, Raymond. *Our Earth Our Cure*. Swan House, 1974.

Lindlahr, Victor H. *You Are What You Eat*. Newcastle Publishing, 1971.

Prensky, Joyce. *Healing Yourself*. 402 Fifteenth Avenue East, Seattle, Washington 98112

Samuels, Mike, and Bennett, Hal. *The Well Body Book*. Random House/Bookworks, 1973.

Thomas, Clayton L., and Davis, F. A. *Tabor's Cyclopedic Medical Dictionary*. 1973.

HERNIA

The following is a simple yet in-depth outline for natural treatment of hernia and hernia-type strains. (EDITOR'S NOTE: *It is specifically for inguinal hernias, which are the most common and occur only in men.*)

Please note, for the maintenance of health and prevention of hernia (disease in general), study and understand the causes, number I A and B.

Contained within the treatment (specifically diet, herbs, body work, and light work) is the key to disease preventive life-style. Happiness and a state of emotional well-being are of utmost importance for both maintenance of health and the rejuvenation of function.

For the most complete healing, follow all steps of the outline. (If there is marked pain or if the treatment does not reduce the swelling, a physician's help should be sought.)

CAUSES AND SYMPTOMS

I. **Causes:**
   A. Weakened intestines due to constipation and/or diarrhea with resulting toxic and weakened condition in surrounding muscles.
   B. Improper lifting of heavy loads, causing further weakening or tearing of abdomen muscles.

II. **Symptoms** (get a competent diagnosis):
   A. Pain upon moving, extending from pelvis to chest generally, or in specific location of hernia.
   B. Intestinal bulge just above pelvis bone where a small portion of intestine is protruding through the muscle.
   C. Intestine can fall into scrotum in severe cases if proper treatment is delayed.
   D. Symptoms can be similar to appendicitis symptoms.

TREATMENT (outline of natural care):

I. **Immediate rest** at first sign (or when you decide to begin your healing).
   A. No lifting.
   B. No strenuous exercise.
   C. Bed rest if severe.

II. **Diet**—to lighten intestinal load and toxic-weakened muscles:
   A. Raw fresh fruits and at least 50 per cent raw vegetables. Fruit and vegetables should not be eaten together. Fresh fruit and vegetable juices could be added to above diet.

(or) B. Fresh raw vegetables and fruit juices i.e.,

carrots	1 lb.
celery	4 stalks
cucumber	1
garlic	5–8 cloves
beet	½ to 1 (with tops)

Drink 1 pint to 1 quart daily, sipped very slowly.

(or) C. Water and tea fast (see III-A).

III. **Herbs:**

A. Tea—to stimulate and strengthen circulation and to cleanse and strengthen bowels, i.e.,

ginger root	1 ounce
fennel seed	1 ounce
buckthorn bark	1 ounce
cayenne	1–2 teaspoons

Mix together. Use 1 heaping teaspoon per cup of boiling water. Steep ½ hour. Drink 2–3 cups daily. Add skullcap or catnip to reduce pain.

B. Poultice: fresh pounded chlorophyll poultice, i.e., comfrey leaves, chickweed, sage, lettuce, watercress, etc.— any one or a mixture. Apply to scrotum (if swollen), pelvis, inguinal (groin), and lower abdomen. Change two or three times daily.

IV. **Body Work:**

A. Massage
1. Entire body. Specifically thighs (insides and outsides), hips, lower back, abdomen, perineum (between anus and genitals), intestine acupoints (gall bladder point on hips).
2. Method: deep muscle, moxa, acumedian, acupressure, or Swedish. Use stimulating oil or liniment.

B. Spinal adjustments
Many times a lumbar misalignment accompanies (or even causes) pain in pelvis, scrotum, or perineum.

C. Slant board
Lie on back 2–3 hours daily, total. It is very important to realign intestines and remove weight from damaged muscles and tissues. Elevate a thinly padded board(s) 18 inches off floor at feet end, with head end on floor.
Follow this order:

1. Abdomen massage—first thing.
2. Rest—i.e., prayer/meditation, sleep, contemplation.
3. Exercise—Lift (as strength allows) one leg at a time, resting often. Eventually work up to both legs lifted. When strength allows, lift both legs, spread apart, down, rest.
4. Rest again.

(NOTE: exercise only on slant board or while lying flat on floor, *not on soft bed*.)

V. Enema—One per day in evenings unless you're eliminating 2–3 times per day. (NOTE: catnip enema or rectum implant useful for relaxation and/or pain relief.)

VI. A hernia belt (available at drugstores) and a male supporter can be beneficial if walking is necessary, but *do not overdo*. Build strength slowly to prevent a relapse (which can be worse and very disheartening).

VII. Light work. The Creator moves within creation as light, animating, healing, loving.

Through prayer, contemplation, meditation our being opens into and fills with light.

A. Some specifics:
   1. Guidance asked and received.
   2. Being is filled with light and peace, reduces stress and shock.
      a. total being.
      b. specific area of disease.
      c. particularly where area is too painful for direct massage.

B. The crux of the situation: faith and focus.

   —from *Mission of Light Notebook* by John Bigler

IMPROVING YOUR HEALTH DURING PREGNANCY

by Harriet Korngold

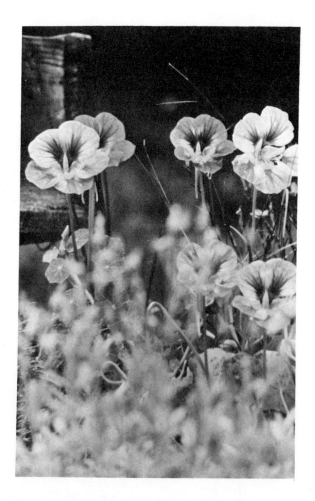

An acupuncturist and former midwife in Peking explains that, according to Chinese medicine, it is the lung energy which holds the fetus in the womb. Oftentimes it is shortly after the onset of a chest cold that either miscarriage or premature birth occurs. The lung energy weakens and the child is released from the womb. It is advised that a woman make sure to take a common cold seriously during pregnancy, get plenty of rest, and drink much comfrey and raspberry leaf tea.

The Chinese say that during delivery the life of the mother is "thin, like paper." After childbirth the woman has a "new life"—she can become healthier and more vigorous than before pregnancy if she pays careful attention, especially the first month after delivery. The kidneys control the reproductive process and are, according to Chinese theory, particularly tired and vulnerable to injury after childbirth. Cold insults the kidney. It is important to avoid any and all cold drinks or foods following delivery and to avoid getting chilled. It is important to keep the low back warm. If the kidneys are insulted at this time, weakness and arthritic symptoms may develop in later life. The Chinese advise the new mother to drink plenty of ginger tea to warm and nourish the blood and to aid in returning the uterus to its former size. Fresh-cooked chicken or chicken broth, simmered with ginger root and dong quai, is good for cleansing and nourishing the blood after birth.

There are many American herbal formulas suggested by Dr. Christopher to be used during pregnancy, delivery, after birth, and for babies and young children.

HERBS THAT HELP DURING PREGNANCY

Red raspberry tea is a powerful astringent which strengthens and tones uterine tissue. It draws iron into the blood and can be used to prevent or treat anemia. Taken regularly throughout pregnancy it will aid in an easy delivery, check hemorrhage during labor, strengthen and cleanse the mucous membranes of the uterus, stomach, and bowels, and enrich the mother's milk. It will help to prevent miscarriage, ease the pain of contractions, and can be used to ease menstrual cramps. For these reasons it is considered to be the classic stand-by herb to be used daily throughout pregnancy.

THE IMPORTANCE OF CALCIUM

The need for calcium is greatly increased during pregnancy and lactation. Sufficient calcium is necessary to insure proper structural development of the child and to protect the bones, teeth, and gums of the mother. If calcium is deficient the child draws what it needs first from the mother's long bones in the leg, creating cramps and leg ache. Calcium is also required for the happy functioning of the kidney. Water retention, varicose veins, and insomnia during pregnancy may all be signs of insufficient calcium. Steel-cut oats soaked overnight and cooked in a double boiler until soft are a good breakfast food, rich in cal-

cium. Molasses and raisins, high in iron, may be added. Sesame butter and figs are also calcium-rich. Vitamin D, obtained from either the sun or cod-liver oil, is necessary for the proper absorption of calcium; magnesium is also needed. There are two powerful formulas for augmenting the calcium obtained from food and may be substituted for drinking milk.

1. 6 organic eggshells
    1 cup apple cider vinegar
    1 cup honey

Crush the eggshells in the solution of vinegar and honey (by hand or in a blender). The calcium is leached by the solution. Take 1 tablespoon 1–3 times each day.

2. 6 parts horsetail grass
    4 parts comfrey
    3 parts oatstraw
    1 part lobelia

Either brew this mixture as a tea (1 ounce of the mixture steeped in 1 pint of water) and take 1 cup 3 times a day *or* use the herbs in powder form, mixed and taken in 2 number 00 capsules 3 times a day.

PREGNANCY PROBLEMS

Nausea or morning sickness is not a normal state to be resigned to during the early phase of pregnancy. It is a sign that the body is lacking in what it requires during this crucial stage when all the basic organs and bony structure are being formed. The B vitamins are especially valuable in overcoming nausea. Ten mg of vitamin B_6 with 50 mg of magnesium, taken 3 times a day, has combated morning sickness for many women within the space of several days. Brewer's yeast will provide the important balance of B vitamins;

take at least 2 tablespoons a day. This will help bring in the breast milk and is also a source of protein. (EDITOR'S NOTE: *Bee pollen can also be taken in juice as a B vitamin supplement.*)

Four hundred mcg of folic acid and 40 mcg of B_{12} along with B_6 can combat anemia as effectively as taking iron supplements without robbing the body of vitamin E. (This happens when taking ferrous sulphate, a type of iron pill often given as a prenatal supplement.) Vitamins C, E, A, and D are also important. Protein, in whatever form, is very necessary to help build the cells and tissue of the complete human being who is being formed. Comfrey tea, the great cell-proliferant, is helpful in this regard. Avoid fried or spicy foods. Plenty of positive, healthy psychic energy, love, fresh air exercise, and natural foods all provide the nourishment so needed at this time.

A valuable formula to correct malpresentations and strengthen the mother for a healthy, easy delivery is Dr. Christopher's "prenatal formula" to be taken only six weeks prior to delivery. It contains pennyroyal, which is an abortive if used earlier in the pregnancy.

Use equal parts:
  false unicorn
  blue cohosh
  pennyroyal
  squaw vine
  holy thistle
  goldenseal
  lobelia

Steep 1 teaspoon per cup of boiling water. Take 1 cup morning and night.

For healthy skin during pregnancy, add ½ cup apple cider vinegar to bath water. The astringent properties of the vinegar are helpful in keeping the vaginal area clean and free from discharge and infection. Massaging the breasts and belly alternately with wheat germ, olive, and castor oil will prevent stretch marks and maintain good skin tone.

HERBS THAT HELP DURING AND AFTER PREGNANCY

To stimulate contractions, use black cohosh tea. Also, rub the acupuncture point located between the bones of the index finger and thumb on the back of the hand. For bleeding during labor use 6 parts false unicorn with 1 part lobelia. To aid in delivery of the placenta use licorice tea. For hemorrhage after birth use black cohosh. To stimulate and augment milk flow use blessed or holy thistle. To improve the quality of milk, add marshmallow root. If mastitis or engorgement of the breast occurs, use a fomentation of 3 parts mullein and 1 part lobelia: brew a strong tea and soak a piece of cotton in the tea and cover the breast, preferably overnight. This formula is good for any glandular swelling.

HERBS FOR BABIES AND CHILDREN

Red raspberry or mullein tea can be used to clear the baby's eyes. For bronchial problems or asthma use 6 parts comfrey and 1 part lobelia as a tea. Use 2 tablespoons 4–5 times a day. For difficult breathing use 1 drop tincture of lobelia in 2 tablespoons peppermint tea. (This dosage is for infants; use ¼–½ cup for older children.) Castor oil and garlic rubbed on the feet is also helpful. For colic, catnip and fennel, peppermint or licorice teas are soothing. If a child will not drink tea it is possible to bathe the baby in a bath with herb tea added. The skin can absorb the benefit of the herbs, especially in children. Linden or lavender flower baths are particularly relaxing. For teething, a good nerve tea to use is 3 parts catnip, 1 part peppermint, 1 part raspberry. The calcium formulas mentioned before are also a great way to ease the discomfort of teething. For diaper rash, powdered slippery elm, comfrey, mullein, and calendula (marigold) can be applied directly. A chickweed bath will also be soothing. For each infection, use 1 drop garlic oil 3 times a day.

_____

All vitamin or mineral supplements referred to should be "organic," derived from plant sources.

TEETHING:

Natural Ways to Turn Cries to Comfort

by Michele Bigler

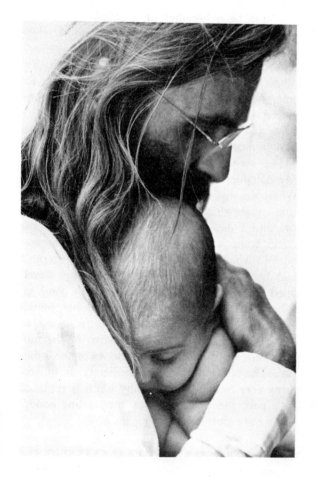

In a hospital emergency room not too long ago were a baby, its mother and grandmother. The baby was feverish and in tears. Talking to the adults and looking at the baby, I discovered that the problems were teething related and the parents hadn't realized it yet. A week later I saw another baby there in the same condition. Again, its parents didn't know what to do to help. (A surgeon informed me that 80 per cent of the hospital's cases could have been handled at home.) This seems to be a fairly common situation. Very often new and experienced parents alike will not realize a child is teething when he or she appears ill.

SOME TEETHING SYMPTOMS

Cheeks will be flushed and the baby will tend to drool a lot. He/she will furiously and intensely suck or chew fingers, thumb, knuckle, blanket, toys, nipples, etc. He/she may bite down hard on an object, pull it out quickly, repeat this motion, and cry. (This hurts if a mother is nursing.) The gums will be tender, swollen, and inflamed. Little ridges begin to push down and up on the gum tissue from inside, and there may be whitish spots on a part of the gums.

It is not uncommon for a normally healthy

baby to develop a cough, fever, runny nose, cold, and/or diarrhea. An otherwise happy baby may fuss and whine, not want to eat, or spit up its food. A baby who would sleep through the night (at last) may become fitful and keep a parent up and down till dawn. Mild skin rashes and diaper rashes are fairly common, as are mild earaches, evidenced by a child pulling or rubbing his/her ear frequently.

GENERAL RELIEF

1 teaspoon chamomile
1 teaspoon peppermint
pinch of hops
2 cups boiling water

Cover and steep. If the pain seems intense add a tiny pinch of lobelia. Serve straight for big kids, dilute for babies.

In a pinch, there is a thing called *"Humphries ⚡3 Homeopathic Preparation for Teething and Wakefulness of Infants."* It contains chamomile, calcium phosphate, coffee, and a trace of belladonna (all in homeopathic—minute—quantities). These are small white balls that pop into the mouth. Drugstores carry them, and they are handy for traveling.

A bit of *eucalyptus oil* rubbed right on the gum helps numb the pain.

Just massaging the gums can bring relief.

FEVER

Add elder flowers and comfrey leaves to the chamo-mint tea, and leave off the hops. Fruit and juices are the best diet at this time. If the child's temperature is severe, a warm peppermint-tea enema works wonders.

Babies begin teething from before three months up to a year. Cutting one tooth can take a week to a couple months from when the first symptoms appear. Symptoms appear on and off, although they are usually worse at night. Between five and seven months the first tooth, most often a lower front, breaks through. This is followed by another next to it, then by either two more bottoms or two tops. Four eyeteeth (the pointed ones), and a set of molars finish the first round. There will normally be a breather of a couple of months, which is a great time for growth and development!

About age two and then again at age six, another set of molars comes in. When looking for emerging teeth, check over the whole mouth. There is no real norm, and it is easy to be fooled. Some children will cut in a "normal" sequence, though most will vary.

The six-year molars can come as a surprise. My daughter is normally a healthy, active child. When she was almost six she developed a recurring cough which went on quite a while. Nothing she and I did seemed to alleviate it. Later she came home with a fever and upset stomach— both of which were gone by the next afternoon. I had forgotten that as a baby she always developed a cough and fever before a tooth came in. When it dawned on me, I checked her mouth and, sure enough, four molars were trying to break through. Within two days two of the molars were in; two weeks later so were the other two. The cough vanished immediately. It still returns very briefly as each baby tooth is replaced by a permanent one, as does "not feeling good." But we are alert to what it means now.

COUGH

If a cough develops, add life everlasting to the chamo-mint. A cough syrup is made by simmering:

1 teaspoon horehound
1 teaspoon slippery elm bark
1 teaspoon mullein
1 teaspoon plantain
2 cups water and lemon juice

Simmer until 2 cups are down to 1 cup; add 1 tablespoon honey. Serve ½–1 teaspoon every couple of hours, depending on the size of the child. If a cough or mucus discharge does develop, cut down on all dairy products and on bread. Lots of vegetables are best.

For *pain, irritability, and sleeplessness in older children,* use ½ cap of powdered valerian, hops, and skullcap, usually sold for better sleep. A pinch of this in the mouth of small ones over six months is good on long, tiring nights. It helps them and you to sleep.

For *rashes* resulting from diarrhea, use wheat germ oil, vitamin E, an aloe vera gel or lotion, or coconut oil.

Some older children get *mild headaches.* A combination of dandelion root, licorice root, and yellow dock root tea is good. Gentle massage to the head and do-in points related to headaches brings relief also.

Earaches are helped by the herb teas, in addition to a tiny amount of lukewarm sesame oil dropped in the ear. Make sure it is only warm. Even better, steep mullein flowers in sesame oil or wheat germ oil in a dark-colored bottle in the sun for 4–5 days. Have it handy.

The peppermint and chamomile tea is good for *babies who won't eat or who spit up.* Juices can help; make sure that grape or carrot juices are diluted, as they seem to be too strong for most babies straight. Feeding applesauce with powdered alfalfa, slippery elm, and bee pollen helps insure that what they eat is nourishing.

CHEWING-ONS

Some things that are good for chewing on are:

Fennel stalks   Take a stalk ¼–½ inch thick, cut it 3–4 inches long. Peel off the outer layer. As the baby chews it aids the stomach and numbs the gums. Some babies will not like the strong taste for long, some will vaguely notice it. Remember that children teethe off and on until two to two and a half and again at six. This is a good one for older kids.

Licorice root   Helps the stomach and throat, numbs the gum, tastes great, and immensely aids fussiness.

Osha root   Good for cough, fever, stomach, and gums. It has a strong spicy taste and is an excellent blood purifier.

TEETHING CRACKERS

Basic ingredients are:

2 cups flour
1 teaspoon oil
½ teaspoon salt
enough water to pull dough away from sides of bowl

Mix and match the flour (whole wheat, corn, rye, oat, rice, buckwheat). Sweeteners not needed. If desired add:

ground sesame seeds for calcium and protein
   1 tablespoon per cup flour
wheat germ for vitamins
   1 tablespoon per cup
and of course—a touch of cinnamon

Mix everything together and knead until ear lobe consistency. Roll out onto floured board until ½ inch thick. Cut into rectangles or roll into finger shapes. Place on lightly oiled cookie sheet. Bake at 350° until crisp, about ½ hour. Big kids like these as munchies, so tuck some away for your teether.

These are other organic things for chewing on:

corncob (after corn is gone)

apple slices (peeled is best if baby can remove skin)

carrot slices (about ½ inch thick)

celery

dried bananas (these are very messy; cool in fridge)

bread sticks

washed pieces of smooth hardwood

seaweed

fingers

toes (baby's own)

beanbags

teething toys filled with water—place in the refrigerator until cool or frozen

cooled washcloths

any small favorite toy that can be cooled

When teething is in earnest, a cup of tea and a time to relax are important for parents as well. Take it. Even if baby has to cry a bit.

In organically minded families (and even in not so minded) I have seen one parent accuse the other of *causing* a baby's apparent illness or fussiness. Diet, energy, state of mind, and a number of related things are usually mentioned as causes. Although excesses of bread, cheese, sugar, etc., do not help matters, neither does being overly upset or nervous. Parents, please be gentle with each other; help instead of hassling. Mothers and fathers need support from each other, single parents can use assistance from friends. Tension between parents over a child's well-being can do more harm than the teething itself will ever do.

This information is meant as a possible guide in some methods that have worked for myself and the children I have worked with. It is not meant as a substitute for professional advice.

It is collected from many years of osmosis from herb books, healing books, healing festivals, herb and naturopathic doctors, mothers (including my own), siblings, and, most important, seven years of my own children, and a few other small ones who have also grown as my knowledge of them has increased.

COPING WITH THE "CROUP"

by Michele Bigler

The fall-winter weather brings with it a potentially serious children's illness commonly called croup. Croup can be a frightening experience for new and old-hat parents alike. Having a son who is prone to bronchial croup, I'd like to share some knowledge and techniques I've learned,

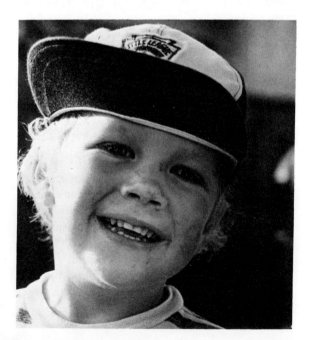

hoping to make it easier for others to use more organic methods to treat it.

Croup is caused by several factors:

1. An excessively heavy diet: i.e., too much bread, dairy, and meat foods, overloading the digestive tract.
2. A contagious viral infection to which the body is made more susceptible by the above.
3. In some children, a food-related allergy.

All of these are complicated by the abrupt weather changes common in late fall and winter. (If you alter your diet from large amounts of fruit to more grains for winter, then back again in the spring, try to concentrate on lots of vegetables during the transition period to avoid extremes that can contribute to contracting diseases.)

Croup often hits unexpectedly at night, in varying degrees. Symptoms are a dry, spasmodic, raspy cough that sounds as if the child is strangling; much difficulty in breathing; bloodshot and/or glazed eyes; fever accompanied by chills. A whistling wheeze on the intake of breath indicates the closing off of the air passages due to swelling and congestion—this is serious. Croup in adults will appear as a laryngitis-type sore throat.

If a child appears flushed and irritated during

the day, with eyes becoming bloodshot or glazed, a hot bath and massage, a tea of peppermint, plantain, and mullein can help offset an attack later. (This can help offset many childhood illnesses.) If coughing is also present, add a ¼ teaspoon dose of goldenseal and some Vicks VapoRub (see recipe for natural vapor rub, page 133) on the chest and back before bed. For very young children, up to a year, cut the amount of goldenseal to ⅛ teaspoon.

If an attack comes at night give an enema of peppermint or catnip tea, and 1 teaspoon strong dandelion tea every couple hours to keep the bowels moving more easily. If you have a vaporizer or humidifier, put a strong tea of mullein, horehound, and lobelia (or any one of these that you have on hand) into it and place the child where he or she can get the most benefit from it. If you do not have either apparatus, fill a bathroom with steam and have the child stay in it breathing as long as possible. Repeat this as often as there is enough hot water. Put horehound and/or mullein tea into a pan on whatever heating system you have and let the house or the room fill up with it. (Keep this going as long as there is difficulty breathing.) A teakettle works well for direction of the steam.

Use vapor rub on the chest and back, and keep the child warm. If breathing is extremely difficult, keep her/him at a 45-degree angle, as the coughing spasms are worse lying down. Mix 1 teaspoon goldenseal with ¼ cup hot water and feed 1 teaspoon every 5–6 hours, or 4 times a day. Make a tea of mullein, yarrow, coltsfoot, and comfrey, and feed it as often and in as much quantity as the child will drink. If there is high fever, add elder blossoms; if the throat has gotten sore, add life everlasting and/or slippery elm. If your child refuses to drink the tea, steep the herbs in apple juice for a while, strain, and serve that way. Sneaky, but effective.

Keep those teas going during the day also. The cough and breathing ease up during the day, and can fool you later. Most croups that I have seen have only one or two bad nights, but you should continue the horehound and mullein for a few days afterwards. Give the goldenseal twice a day, tapering down to once a day when the breathing is normal again.

Diet should consist of fruits and fruit juices for a couple days, with some seaweed-vegetable broth. Especially while fever is present, juices are important. Dehydration can occur, and the throat becomes quite tender. Push the child to drink; many will not want to. Add steamed vegetables, vegetable juices, and tofu for a few days. Keep strictly away from breads, cheeses, eggs, and sugar for a while. Add corn meal cereal and well-cooked millet before adding any type of heavier grain.

One thing . . . Don't be afraid to use the hospital if you feel you want or need to. The hospital uses a small resuscitator with a nose-mouth mask. It force breathes with the child, a full breath of medicated vapor, that clears and opens the air passages. This is a fifteen-minute treatment that could prevent a lot of trauma and pain in severe cases.

Do what you can organically, but if you reach the end of your limit, or the child is not responding to treatment fast enough to prevent suffocation, you can use the medicated vapor treatment, and then continue the herbs, diet, steam with more effectiveness.

Not all cases of croup are serious, but all cases indicate a potential seriousness. I hope this will help parents to deal with it, and ease the worry that I know comes with the croup.

Vapor-rub-type Salve

instructions by Rosemary Gladstar

1. Heat together *gently:*
    1 cup vegetable oil
    ¼ cup beeswax
2. (Take 1 tablespoon of this, remove it from the heat, and let it cool. Test its consistency.) Add more wax if too thin, more oil if too thick.
3. Once you are sure you have the consistency you want, add *drop by drop:*
    eucalyptus oil
    wintergreen oil
    rosemary oil
    lavender oil
    CAUTION: these oils are strong. Smell as you add them. The salve should smell stronger than you want it to be when it has been cooled (you can always reheat and add more oil if it's not strong enough).
4. Pour into jar and allow to cool.

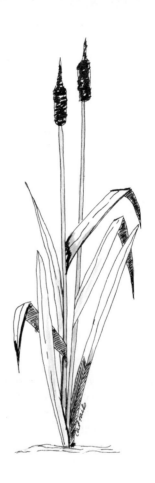

WHAT YOU CAN DO ABOUT CYSTS

by Laura Burns

You're taking a shower, and you feel a lump—first in your breast, then in your throat! Maybe you notice some lumps under your arms also. Before panic sets in, take a deep breath and just sit down. Give yourself a good hug and a kiss and then find out what's happening.

Let's call these lumps cysts—what are they and how are they caused? Cysts are space-occupying lesions and frequently mimic tumors. They usually have fluid contents and are commonly caused by blockage of the ducts in glandular structures (e.g., breasts) or distention of structures having no ducts (ovaries).

Cysts in the breasts are not inflammatory and are probably hormonal in origin. During normal cyclical changes in the ovary, the alternating estrogen and progesterone secretions produce effects in the breasts (so notice if the lumps decrease or disappear fully after you begin menstruating). During the cycle there is an overgrowth of both epithelium and stroma, which return to normal at the end of each cycle. As a result of hormonal imbalance, either the epithelium or stroma or both may remain in an abnormal proliferated state to produce nodular, granular, lumpy, or cystic breasts. These benign growths may occur at any age following puberty.

HERBS

To assist your body a good tea that will affect and balance the glandular-hormonal system will be helpful. The lymphatics and blood will need to be cleansed as well.

Drink 3–4 cups of this tea daily for at least one full cycle. You will probably need to take it longer, though. Use 1 tablespoon/1 cup boiling water. Steep 20–30 minutes. (Make enough to last for a few days, and keep it refrigerated.)

1 part red clover blossoms—excellent lymphatic cleanser—especially for right side of the body (acute conditions)

1 part holy thistle—tonic, cleanses blood, especially good for the female system.

1 part Siberian ginseng—balances out all glandular systems

2 parts sarsaparilla—excellent blood and lymph cleanser. Stimulates estrogen in the body. Acts as a tonic

2 parts Tang Kuei or angelica root—good for all female disorders, vitamin E balancing to system

2 parts echinacea—alterative to the system

3 parts skullcap—tonic and builder to nervous system.

3 parts raspberry leaves—relaxes and aids assimilation of iron and magnesium into the blood

3 parts blue vervain—eliminative to blood, good herb for women strengthening psychically

3 parts blue vervain*

3 parts cramp bark—balances out the ovaries, calms the nerves surrounding them. Acts as an antispasmodic

3 parts holy thistle

DIET

Diet can add to quicker results. Cleansing food would be good. Purple grapes, grape juice, carrots, lots of greens. All of your blue-violet foods would be excellent, such as plums, seaweeds, blueberries, etc. Remember, though—don't restrict yourself too much so that you feel frustrated. It's not so much what you put in your mouth—but what comes out!

THE OVARIES

Some of the symptoms of an ovarian cyst are:
very irregular menses—spaced far and few between or flooding for long periods of time
cramping
weakness

Many people feel that if there is a cyst on the ovary, conception will not be possible. I have known women who have been diagnosed as having an ovarian cyst and became pregnant anyway.

For cysts on the ovaries the tea is similar with a couple of changes:

1 part red clover blossoms

1 part raspberry leaves

1 part Siberian ginseng

2 parts astragalus root—tones the lymphatic system

2 parts pipsissewa—excellent herb for any disorder in the uterine system

2 parts Tang Kuei or angelica root

COLOR

Some color breathing exercises will also be helpful. Just as the sound vibrations of beautiful music can help us to better health, so can the vibrations of colors. They are very simple to do: Picture from within your inner eye a golden rose color—create an image, a smell, whatever—and breathe it in. Feel it slowly fill up your entire being until you experience a beautiful "rosy glow." Then wash yourself with a blue-violet color. Again picture this blue-violet light—place it on top of your head. As you inhale, bring that color down through your crown and out your toes. Do this a couple of times and see if you don't feel a bit more refreshed. (The combinations of the above herbs reflect a rose-violet vibration.) Just as wearing our favorite color is uplifting and comforting, wearing these particular colors mentally mobilizes our own healing forces to correct the imbalances.

CHANGE

The breasts and the entire pelvic region are two very powerful creative centers in the body. (The breasts are full of pyramidal shaped lobules!) Take a good personal inventory of what may be blocking your expression. Love, accept, and work with yourself. Disharmonies in the body just reflect old habit patterns, waiting to be changed by a clear, loving attitude.

* If you are experiencing menstrual flooding, substitute lady's mantle.

GETTING OFF THE PILL

by Laura Burns

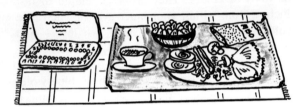

Most medical doctors will agree that it takes a woman's hormonal system up to two years to "recover" after the birth-control pills are stopped. The Pill alters the functioning of the pituitary gland—a very important gland of the body. This gland's main physical function is to secrete hormones which regulate the activity of various organs of the body. The two hormones directly affecting ovulation are follicle stimulating hormone (FSH) and luteinizing hormone (LH). The pituitary also secretes a hormone which affects fat and carbohydrate metabolism (GH). An upset of this hormone is one reason why some people have uncontrolled weight gain. Other hormones secreted by the pituitary are: ACTH, which affects the adrenal cortex, a thyroid-stimulating hormone, an antidiuretic hormone which affects the kidneys in their reabsorption of water into the blood, and oxytocin which stimulates contractions in the uterus and promotes lactation (milk production). *Use of the Pill, with its profound effect upon pituitary functions, means more than just birth-control "safety."*

It has been found that birth-control pills cause certain vitamin deficiences—B, iron, and folic acid (vitamin M). The B vitamins have a lot to do with nervousness, depression, faulty metabolism, and pernicious anemia. Folic acid strengthens the capillary walls and intestines and prevents anemia. Iron builds and strengthens the blood, allowing the transport of oxygen to the cells.

If you have taken the Pill for any length of time it would be beneficial to tone up your whole system. Some good sources for folic acid are fresh mushrooms, leafy vegetables, and dried dates. (Please note that when vegetables are stored at room temperature much of the folic acid is lost.) Some of the red and purple fruits and vegetables are great for iron—such as beets, black figs, miso, seaweeds, molasses, and watercress (which is classified as a "red" vegetable). For the B vitamins, wheat sprouts, bee pollen, rice bran syrup, seeds, nuts, dairy products, brewer's yeast, etc.

A good herbal tonic is also advisable. The following tea will help to stimulate and normalize the hormonal-glandular system and build and strengthen the blood and the kidneys:

yellow dock root—high in vitamins and trace minerals and builds up the blood

nettle leaves—high in iron and builds and strengthens the kidneys

Siberian ginseng—stabilizes the glandular system

false unicorn root—stimulates the production of estrogen

sarsaparilla—stimulates the production of estrogen

cramp bark—balances the ovaries

Tang Kuei—Chinese herb, helps to normalize the entire uterine system

These are all equal parts by weight. If the Siberian ginseng herb cannot be found, the extract can be used by adding it to the tea. At least two cups should be drunk per day for at least a month. This will hasten your body to return to normal.

STAYING LOOSE WITH MENSTRUAL CRAMPS

by Denni McCarthy

Long ago I realized that nothing comes to me by accident. When I feel pain I try to discover why. Sometimes the answer is elusive, but ultimately it takes me within myself. I had always been one of those fortunate women who rarely had cramps, until two years ago. I was on my way up a long, bumpy, mountainous road in Costa Rica when I became weak, nauseated, and hopelessly cramped. Stopping in the shade for a few hours and deep breathing relieved me. Since then I've been working to bring my system back into balance and to deal with monthly cramps.

RELAXING RELIEVES CRAMPS

Dysmenorrhea is the official name for those painful spasms of the uterus. Cramps sounds more like the actual experience. Some theories suggest it's activated by a hormonal imbalance. Whatever the actual biological cause there's a lot you can do to work with your discomfort. One of the primary things is to RELAX. Give yourself the space and time to lie down. Keep warm and breathe deeply into your uterus. Visualize it as free from pain and totally let go of any tension. Some women find a heating pad helpful. I've found too much heat increases the flow and the pain—especially too many hot baths. Another woman has used ginger slices over her pelvic area covered with a hot towel. Most important is to allow yourself to do nothing for as long as it takes the cramps to pass.

HERBAL HEALING

There are many herbal aids for cramps. Pennyroyal (squaw mint) tea is the most effective for me. I just steep 1 teaspoon of the dried herb in 1 cup boiled water for 10 to 20 minutes, drink it, and lie down. In about ½ hour my cramps are usually gone. I've used chamomile, cramp bark, rosemary, and valerian in the same manner as pennyroyal. One cup taken daily for 5 days before my period is due has often brought relief from cramps. These herbs help to tone the female organs and bring them back into a comfortable balance. Footbaths with pennyroyal are especially soothing, the warmth penetrating and relaxing the whole body. I also made a small pillow stuffed with dried pennyroyal flowers (dried leaves will work too) that I keep by me during the heaviest pain; the energy transmitted by them is very healing. Always remember to use these herbs with caution, utilizing minimal amounts depending on your own requirements.

EXERCISE—YOGA

There are several body postures that help tone the uterus and relieve pain. One is to simply curl up into a tight fetal position. Another is the Fallen Leaf, in which you pull your knees to your chest, your cheek on the floor, and your arms stretched out beside you or tucked underneath.

I find that bending over in a cross-legged position with my forehead touching the ground helps. Other women have said that the Cobra and back bends stretch out the area and minimize the pain.

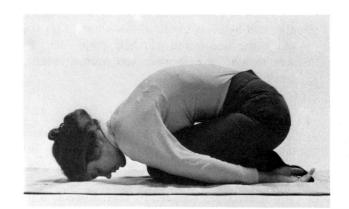

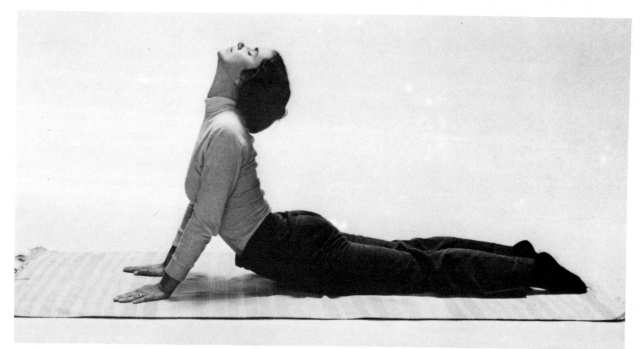

FRIENDS CAN HELP

A friend can give you the space you need to be alone and relax. If you want closeness, then a cup of tea, a light massage, or just warm hands can do wonders. It seems that men also have their cycles, and by being aware of this natural fact you can better understand and help each other. Be sure to ask for help when you want it; even a small act can be healing.

DIET

Your diet in relation to menstruation is important. Constipation can have a lot to do with cramps, so eat a few prunes or figs or drink senna leaf tea to keep your bowels loose. Calcium is also needed. It's supplied by sesame seeds, comfrey, dairy products, and lemons. Iron is often depleted at this time; it's found in molasses, apricots, eggs, milk, and whole grains. Vitamin C will help your body to assimilate the iron. Foods high in vitamins E and B can also be used. I like to fast when my cramps are the worst, drinking fresh carrot, cucumber, and parsley juice or just pennyroyal tea. Remember to eat lightly and listen to what your body demands.

Cramps are incredible teachers and can guide you toward looking at your whole being. Ask yourself, "What have I been eating? Have I been exercising? Have I been positive? Have I been tense?" An answer to these things can give you clues about what's going on within and move you into helping yourself through cramps.

(EDITOR'S NOTE: *Some people find valerian nauseating. If you wish to try it, first drink a small amount. If it doesn't seem to bother you, you can take more.*)

MENOPAUSE:

It's Not in Your Mind, It's in Your Body

by Carole Johnson

If you are forty-five or so you are already familiar with the symptoms of menopause. Each
month your period may be accompanied by
blinding headaches, the feeling that you are having a severe attack of flu or some such disease.
Anger and frustration well up unexpectedly, old
friends, children, husbands seem to be enemies.
The whole world is against you and you are cry-
ing. What a picture! Twenty-five per cent of
women have these symptoms as well as the usual
hot flashes that are the subject of so many jokes.
The rest have other assorted effects like muscle
cramps, heart palpitations, exhaustion, and some
not invented yet. Yet menopause is not thought
of as a disease. If your doctor is willing to talk to
you about it at all (I'm from the east) he will tell
you that happy, well-adjusted women don't have
these symptoms (what does that make you?),
and that you should go home and be happy, ignore your condition, and if you're lucky, maybe
two, three, or ten years later it will go away. Two
or three years later many women are hospitalized
for nervous breakdown, others have lost their be-
wildered husbands, their figures, the love of their
children, their self-respect, and their ability to
work. Let me ask you, what is there left?

I WOULDN'T ACCEPT IT

Because of the unique profession I am in (I am
an art therapist), when my turn came, I was not
willing to accept the "it's all in your mind" excuse
for lack of adequate medical information. I knew
my mind and it had been more free, stronger, and
happier than it had ever been when those first un-
expected symptoms hit. I was sure I had the
Asian flu. The second time I thought I was being
poisoned by something in the environment,
which, in a way, I was, and the third time I went
to the doctor. Three periods in a row was too
much of a coincidence. He suggested a psychiatrist and some hormones because of the severity
of the symptoms. I talked to a friend who was a
psychiatrist and who knew me well, just to cover
all the bases. We agreed to look elsewhere. If it
wasn't all in the mind, what and where was it?

THE SEARCH

I started interviewing other women. They were
as much in the dark as the doctors. I finally
found a good book on the subject. It was written
by a woman with the same experience who had
taken it upon herself to gather all the information
on menopause she could find. I was now well in-

formed as to symptoms and expectations (all bad) but nothing on relief beyond a strong will and lots of endurance. My headaches turned into migraines (suspiciously psychosomatic), sometimes eight days' worth. When I was out of the dope long enough, I found a book on migraine. One sentence stood out for me. Among all the emotional stress reasons for migraine was the fact that sometimes undigested proteins in the blood cause this headache. Next I researched stress, digestion, and ultimately nutrition. I had gained thirty pounds and had so much gas in my intestine I had given up visiting friends. Eventually the nutrition books led me to the International Association for Cancer Victims and Friends, where I found a whole new approach to health—natural food healing. I went on an eight-day fast (juice, fruit, and enemas). Immediately, I lost eight pounds. I began eating raw foods (*"live,"* in the lingo), salads, sprouts, nuts, and lots of carrot juice, organic if possible. The next month I cut my headache medication in half. Four months later I was off all pills including hormones and tranquilizers (I'd been on these for seven years), and I was down to a beautiful 120 pounds. I still had about ten pretty tired miserable days each month but I was enough better to know I was on the right track!

I have a long way to go to repair the damage that was done these last three years but the joy is that it can be repaired and the information passed on to others.

WHAT REALLY HAPPENS

At menopause the whole body system is temporarily out of balance. If all the glands and organs are healthy, just reducing the digestive load and staying away from salt and animal protein for a while would probably be enough therapy. However, most of us have been overeating meat and salt for years, have damaged livers and kidneys (our detoxifiers) from X ray, chemically treated water, smog, coal-tar-based medications (contraceptive pills), food additives, DDT, and other pesticides in our food, as well as impaired digestive tracts from refined, processed (dead), and cooked foods. With a limping metabolic system, food is not digested or assimilated, the body starves and feels exhausted. Overeating to relieve exhaustion causes toxins to build up in the body and fluids to be stored in the tissues, with the accompanying accelerated weight gain. The period with its natural stresses and metabolic changes becomes an overload for the glandular and nervous system. You are now suffering from malnutrition, autotoxemia (self-poisoning), and understandable exhaustion, with all the painfully real symptoms of a disease which it is. This is a perfect physical climate to accept degenerative diseases, like cancer, arthritis, arteriosclerosis, etc. You deserve a better fate than this!!!! I am now forty-eight, eat 75 per cent raw foods, drink detoxification herb teas and liver extracted broth (which by the way is delicious). I fast on juice and fruit two days before my period. When toxins build up (menopausal symptoms) I take a coffee enema to relieve the pain. (Read about this in Max Gerson's *Cancer Therapy—50 Cases*). I am able to sit in the sun again, have no more dripping nose, watery-eyed allergies (an interesting point that needs looking into), I am taking tennis lessons, wear a two-piece bathing suit, and am getting my master's degree.

YOU TOO CAN FEEL THIS GREAT!

It's not all in your mind—it IS in your body!!!

Get it all out with a natural, organic detoxification diet. Take your life in your own hands! What have you got to lose?

CLEARING:

A Home Guide to Better Relationships

by David Copperfield

Have you ever let some little thing irk you so long that you "blew your stack"? Have you ever known anyone who would let difficulties build up with others to the point where someone would have to leave? We all know that repressing emotions helps to cause ulcers, high blood pressure, and upset stomach, as well as headaches. Talk to almost any runaway and you'll find "We just couldn't communicate." On the other hand constant emotional outbursts, nagging, and nitpicking are a drag.

There is a better way. Out of modern psychology, interest in self-awareness, the desire to love one another, and plain old COMMON SENSE comes the practice known as CLEARING.

WHAT IS CLEARING?

Clearing is walking up to someone and saying "I have something that I need to clear up with you . . . would now be good or later?" Very simple words that sometimes take a lot of courage to say. Clearing is letting another person know anything that may be clogging the lines of communication between you. It is putting such value on your relationship and the feeling of clarity between you that you are willing to express even *petty* feelings that are hassling you. Clearing is choosing honesty over convenience. Although keeping clear with people takes a certain portion of one's time, the results are usually increased efficiency on all levels—your own mind is clearer; and work that demands co-operation flows much smoother. Clearing is caring enough to say the very worst in a loving and honest way.

WHAT IT ISN'T

Many times John will tell Philip that he's being unfair, selfish, and too noisy. Philip, feeling that he's being fair under the circumstances, will argue the point. This is an example of what clearing isn't. It isn't telling another person about himself, i.e.: "You're this way, you're that way." Clearing *is* telling another how their actions made you feel—like "When you came in and turned on the radio, I felt interrupted—I felt irritated when I lost track of what I was working on." In clearing, all you are doing is expressing *your feelings*. You are not making a judgment.

ROUGH BEGINNINGS

At first I found it hard to clear but I was working with someone who wanted to practice it. This helped a lot. It gave me confidence and experience for attempts to clear with others on my own initiative. It did take courage to walk up to someone and say that there was something that needed to be cleared between us. I got more courage and felt more relaxed about it as I practiced it more and more. As I cleared up one level of irritation, there often appeared another, less conscious, level. I was getting in touch with stuff that affected me but that I was unaware of before. I also found that it was good to be conscious of whether the other person was in a good place and space for clearing. I'd simply tell him/her I had something to clear and ask if now would be good or later. (One couple I know has a special candle

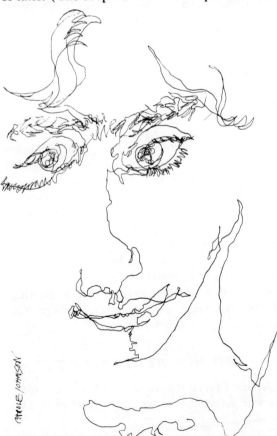

they received as a wedding present which one or the other lights when there is a difficulty that must be talked out. The candlelight tends to soften the atmosphere and symbolizes bringing problems to Light.)

THE PROCESS UNFOLDS

This is a formula for a clearing session. Each step is an important part of the process. After doing it a few times the process will just be "second nature" to you.

1. Find a private place that seems comfortable to both of you.

2. Sit in a relaxed position facing each other. Be close enough to hold hands. Sometimes touching helps, but at other times it may be impossible until after clearing.

3. Take a few deep breaths together to relax and center yourselves. Let go of other concerns and be right there.

4. One person begins by telling his feelings, what he has been experiencing and is experiencing right now. The listener should just listen, not think of answers or *alibis,* not build a defense. Just let the speaker air his feelings.

5. After the feelings of one have been aired, the other gets a chance to do the same. Avoid interrupting one another to correct certain views. The feelings are more important than accuracy of details.

6. Let each other's feelings affect you. Tell each other how they make you feel. Remember, you each have a "right" to feel the way you do and you each have a responsibility to accept the truth.

7. You'll feel a lifting of the tension after a while if you've both searched your hearts and voiced every emotion. The space between you will begin to feel clear again. Remind each other

to keep clear—don't let feelings build up, but clear each little irritation as it happens.

Sometimes it helps to have a third person present who also understands clearing, who can act as a "referee." This person can make sure that one of the clearers doesn't keep "hedging" or interrupting the other. He can make sure both participants are expressing their *feelings* rather than opinions or projections. He must only "butt in" when it's necessary and not add his advice or opinions to help one or the other. He must be an honest observer that both clearers respect.

ASKING FOR HELP

When requesting a difficult clearing session I could approach it by saying that I was having some bad feelings and needed help with them. When I ask for another's help in changing *my* state of mind, they're usually willing to even change a little themselves, to help me.

Realizing that it's *my* feelings that are the problem and not totally the actions of another places a new perspective on human relations. Clearing can be embarrassing—the ego may seem to suffer a bit—but valuing a relationship will make one willing to hazard it. Two wonderful by-products will occur as time goes on; a clearer understanding of your own nature and feelings and a growing perception of the clarity between yourself and others.

Clearing is *caring enough* to say the very worst in an honest and loving way.

GROUP CLEARING: WORKING IT OUT TOGETHER

In any group there are bound to be disagreements, from basic personality conflicts to petty friction. Like it or not, we humans walk a rocky road trying to work together.

Many kinds of groups can use Group Clearing . . . families, working groups, businesses, and anyone involved in group experiences such as clinics, community gardens, and school staffs. By making Group Clearing the most important meeting of the week your group may find, as we have, that other meetings become less needed.

Group Clearing allows us to share on deep levels so people understand why we act as we do. It lets everyone in the group (not just our close friends) in on ourselves. Folks who practice group clearing begin to see themselves more clearly as individuals and as group members.

It must be admitted that it takes a certain amount of courage to jump into Group Clearing just as it does to use individual clearing.

YOU CAN CO-ORDINATE YOUR GROUP CLEARING

Someone needs to step forward to suggest and guide the first few Group Clearing sessions. Here's a step-by-step plan that you can use.
1. Pick the best time for the most people.
2. Create a comfortable setting with some sort of seating arrangement in which everyone can see everyone else in your group.
3. Get things warmed up by sharing an experi-

ence together. Perhaps a song, holding hands for a minute or two, or just a brief period of silence. The idea is to get people focusing on the group.

4. Now suggest that everyone who wishes to, one by one, share where they are. You can start, thereby giving others a chance to see how to do it. Tell how you are doing physically, spiritually, and emotionally (any or all). Second, try to relate your inner experience to your outer actions in work, relating, and attitudes. And finally, if you have some feelings you need to express to someone in your group, this is the time to do it.

    First: share where you are in your inner life.
    Second: tie that together with how you've been acting and functioning.
    Third: clear with anyone if a block comes to mind.

You may find it easiest to use a "talking stick" (any handy object) that identifies the speaker. This is handed on by each speaker in turn.

5. Allow pauses to occur between speakers. This lets everyone digest what was just said. If someone starts right away, that's O.K. too.
6. When everyone who wants to has shared once, then you can let various people express feelings and reactions. Use the "talking stick" if it feels right but be looser about it.
7. When everyone seems to have shared and cleared, suggest a blessing and unifying process.
    Perhaps a prayer: asking for clarity throughout the week.
    Perhaps a meditation: feel yourself as an individual and also as a member of the group. Hold the thought of thankfulness for clarity.
    Sing a song together: be joyful, be thankful.
    Form a foot rub circle: on the floor or sitting in chairs in a circle. Suggest everyone extend his/her right foot to the person on the right. Start with the calf and work to the toes and then back down to the heel.
    Hold hands and be silent together: Try one of these or a combination of one or all. We like them all and do them at random before, during, and after Group Clearing.

GETTING CLEAR

Remind yourself and the group that there may be a period of tension when personal and group blocks begin to surface, but that a great feeling of relief, clarity, and unity will naturally follow. The next morning and the following days will undoubtedly be affected. After a good rain, the air is fresh and the flowers glisten. Group Clearing is for people much like the rain is for plants.

Concentrate on sharing and clearing up what you experienced last week . . . or what you are experiencing in the moment . . . avoid going back much further into the past unless it is greatly affecting the present.

INTERRUPTING THE PROCESS

During your meeting someone may feel "unclear" or "hassled" by something being said (for example the person speaking is talking too long and someone feels bored). Suggest that anyone feeling uncomfortable stop the process (with the O.K. of the present speaker) and tell how what's being said is making him/her feel. Like, "You know, I agree with the ideas you're expressing but the vibrations you're putting with them really make me feel uncomfortable." Then you can discuss the vibrations together. You can explore why they made you feel bad—what buttons the vibrations pushed in you. And the other member can try to see what was causing the vibrations—why the vibrations got linked up with the ideas being talked about.

Both folks should then be clearer and have learned a bit more about themselves and their own reactions. Then you can suggest, if necessary, that the process continue.

KEEPING CLEAR

Agree to clear problems right away whenever possible.

Agree to try to clear alone with the person you experience a problem with. If it isn't working out, find someone to remain neutral and assist the two of you in clearing. If it is still not working, bring the problem before the whole group.

Agree to listen to a person completely before responding. Listen to his/her emotions. Try not to get bogged down in specific complaints, but respond from your heart and emotions. Clear how that made you feel rather than argue about who is right and who is wrong.

It may help to remember that no one meeting is all-important. The first meeting may be very uneventful. But you can bet that even if folks aren't speaking up, there's still a lot going on inside them. Each Group Clearing seems to have a cumulative effect. And it gets easier as time goes on.

INTERESTING THINGS TO NOTE

We've gotten so we look forward to our Group Clearing (most of the time). People who haven't found time for our meetings have tended to drop out of our business family. For us, working closely requires clarity. One side effect is that work gets done more efficiently. For instance, fewer people are needed to make specific decisions as we become surer of the motives of others. People seem relieved and happy after a Group Clearing.

We have begun meeting right after work (5 P.M.) on Tuesdays, going at it for about three hours and then sharing a light soup and salad together. The "fast" aids the clearing and the meal helps us get used to the new relationships we've just discovered in each other. Meeting early in the week helps the rest of the week go smoothly. Wednesday really feels CLEAR.

Clearing is caring enough to say the very worst in an honest and loving way. Its practice will make you clearer about yourself, and that's the first step in understanding others. It may be hard at first and take more courage than you think you can muster, but I'm sure you'll find it's well worth it.

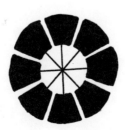

HERB PREPARATIONS

POTENT POTIONS

by Rosemary Gladstar

Learning to use herbs is a challenging adventure. When combined in harmonious patterns, herbs become powerful, gentle medicine. Teas, tonics, salves, and liniments are preparations you can make yourself. Learn basic recipes and harmonious combinations of herbs. As your knowledge of these healing plants expands you'll know better which herbs work best together.

In preparing medicinal teas, potency and harmony are most important. Many herbs are recommended for each disease; however, there are usually a few herbs which combine most effectively to combat the illness. Learning which herbs are most effective is the duty of the herbalist. By using several reference herbals and cross-checking herbs and illnesses, by talking to others who use herbs as medicine, and especially by drawing upon your own experience, your knowledge of the healing power of herbs will rapidly expand.

BASIC TEA PREPARATION

Herbal teas may be taken internally or used externally as poultices, fomentations (applications of hot and cold water), or in baths to purify and relax the body. To prepare leaves, flowers and stems, add 1 teaspoon of herb to 1 cup boiling hot water. Let steep 15–20 minutes, keeping covered. Strain and use. Roots, seeds, and bark must be

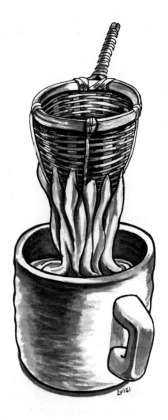

simmered (low boil) at least 15 minutes; keep pan covered; strain and use. When using internally remember: ¼ cup of herbal medicine taken several times during the day is far better than 2 cups gulped down at once.

COUGH SYRUP

Teas are but one way to prepare herbs as medicine. Herbal syrups are very effective for coughs and sore throats. Easy to prepare, too. Use 2 ounces of your chosen herb blend to 1 quart of water. Simmer slowly, keeping pan covered, until liquid is reduced to ½. Strain and add 1½ cups honey. Simmer a few minutes until syrup thickens. Remove from heat and carefully add 1 or 2 drops of peppermint oil (the oil is very strong, so be careful how much you add). An excellent cough syrup consists of

slippery elm bark
fennel seeds
wild cherry bark   } equal parts
licorice root
sweet orange peel
or
coltsfoot
comfrey   } equal parts
mullein
lobelia (¼ part)

You'll find each of these herbs has been used through the ages for sore throats, cough, and mucus discharge.

LINIMENTS

Often, herbs render their essence more readily to alcohol than to water. Powerful liniments can be prepared using an alcohol, witch hazel, or vinegar base. Liniments are used externally to disinfect, heal wounds, cure poison oak and other skin infections and aid in soothing sore muscles. Steep 3 ounces powdered or granulated herb in astringent base at least 7 days. Keep in covered glass container in a sunny window or warm spot and shake every day. Strain the liquid, label container, and store in a cool place.

My favorite liniment is prepared of:

2 ounces myrrh gum powder
2 ounces goldenseal powder
¾ ounce cayenne powder

Steep in 1 quart rubbing alcohol at least 1 week. Strain and keep in airtight glass container. A very effective remedy for open wounds (it stings), skin infections such as poison oak, boils, pimples, and offers some relief for sore muscles.

SALVES

Herbal salves are another useful preparation to make. Many of the wild herbs found growing make effective wound salves: chickweed, plantain, dock, comfrey, burdock, to mention a few. To prepare, take 1 cup pure vegetable oil, 1–2 ounces beeswax, and 1–2 ounces of herb. Vitamin E oil is optional. If using granulated herbs, let herb sit overnight (or longer) in oil. Slowly simmer herb in oil 15–20 minutes. Strain and add 1 ounce beeswax to herbal oil. Stir until wax is melted. Let cool in pan and add additional beeswax if needed. Reheat and pour into salve container. If using powdered herbs, heat slowly in oil 15 minutes and add wax. Test the texture by letting the mixture cool in a spoon. If needed, add more wax. Stir frequently while salve cools as the powdered herbs tend to settle to the bottom. When nearly cooled, spoon into salve containers. The salves used most in my work are goldenseal salve and St. John's salve, both excellent preparations for open sores, infections, and burns.

GOLDENSEAL SALVE

1 ounce goldenseal powder
1 ounce myrrh gum powder
Vitamin E oil

Prepare as above for powdered herbs.

ST. JOHN'S SALVE

½ ounce St. John's wort
½ ounce marigold flowers
Vitamin E oil

Prepare as above for whole herbs.

HERBAL BATHS

Perhaps the simplest way to enjoy the pleasure of herbs is bathing amongst them. In the warmth of a bath the water opens the pores, allowing the entire body to drink of the plants' essence. This simple luxury may be enjoyed by all. If you haven't a bath, facial steams and footbaths make a satisfying substitute.

There are several methods for preparing herbs for the bath and many combinations to play with. One way is to tie herbs in a muslin or cheesecloth bag and secure onto tub faucet. By allowing only hot water to run for the first few minutes, you extract the relaxing essences. Adjust the water temperature, untie the bag from the faucet, and use as a tonifying scrub over your entire thirsting body. For fragrant ecstasy combine:

½ cup each of
  chamomile
  lavender
  rose petals
  spearmint

OR

½ cup each of
  orange flowers
  comfrey leaf
  lemon verbena
  roses or lavender

Prepare as above, or steep herbs in 2 quarts water for 20 minutes. Strain and add liquid to bath water.

HOMEMADE SOAPS

If you feel you must use soap, make your own. Grate a bar of pure castile soap into a bowl. Have ready chamomile or comfrey tea and add just enough to soap flakes to create a thick paste. Work in oatmeal, almond meal, and a bit of gum benzoin powder. Knead until you get the consistency of thick bread dough. You may want to add a favorite scent or, for dry skin, apricot or almond oil. Roll into balls or fashion fancy shapes. Allow to harden a couple of days.

For deep pore cleansing, combine equal parts almond meal, oatmeal flour, and corn meal. Store in a jar by the sink. To use, moisten a small amount with water or honey and massage into face. Rinse with warm water.

AFTERSHAVE LOTION

This is wonderfully cooling and refreshing.
1 pint witch hazel or
      rubbing alcohol or
      apple cider vinegar
a couple of ounces of each in equal proportions:
  sage
  rosemary
  mint
Combine ingredients and let sit 7–14 days in a closed glass container. Shake daily. After a week or two, strain out the herbs and add a *tiny* bit of wintergreen or peppermint oil and shake to distribute. If you use vinegar dilute the tincture with a little rose water.

BODY OILS

Body oils are another of nature's pleasures so simple to prepare. Lavender, chamomile, comfrey, elder, patchouly, raspberry, rosemary, chickweed, sage, mints, lemon verbena, orange peels and flowers are among the plants which best benefit your skin. Place herbs in a widemouthed glass jar and cover with almond or apricot oil, being certain the herb is covered by two or three inches of oil. Add 10,000 I.U. vitamin E oil. (This acts as a preservative.) Let sit in a warm place for three weeks. Strain well through cheese-cloth. The oil will be deeply infused with the essence of flowers and leaves, but often is not as sweetly scented as you may wish. A drop or two of your favorite scent is all that is needed.

There is little mystery in the beauty one gains from nature's gifts. Immersing ourselves in her full-bodied beauty, we become a clear pool of reflection.

HOW TO PREPARE AND USE
COMPRESSES, POULTICES, AND FOMENTATIONS

These are common external treatments that have been used throughout the ages to relieve pain and promote healing. They should always be accompanied by appropriate internal treatments.

A compress is the application of moist heat or cold to a specific area of the body to enhance healing. It can be used over a poultice or by itself. Its moisture helps its effectiveness.

To prepare a compress place a thin towel over the area you will be working on to absorb excess moisture. Have the hot or ice-cold water ready (see below for when to use hot or cold compress). Keep the hot water covered as much as possible to prevent it from cooling too quickly. Fold a washcloth in half, then in half again so you have a long, thin cloth. Holding by the ends dip it into the water, hold it there a few moments, then lift it and wring it out thoroughly, using both hands. (If you are using hot water this could be painful, so while the cloth is in the water dip your hand into very cold water, then wring quickly. You won't feel the heat as much.) Apply the compress over the towel. Leave the compress on until it begins losing its warmth or coldness.

When to use a compress sprains—cold compress (ice bag) initially; after healing begins use alternating hot and cold. Headache, inflamed jaw—cold compress. To draw out poisons—hot infusion of yerba santa. Aching joints—mugwort, stinging nettle. Swollen glands—hot infusion of mullein.

A poultice is any substance applied to the body for healing. Mud, bread, baking soda, and various plants are among the substances which have been used on the body for specific reasons.

To prepare a poultice mash, masticate, crush, etc., to make the substance into a paste, using warm water or apple cider vinegar if necessary. Cover the affected area with a thin piece of muslin, then apply substance. Tape or bandage it into place. Change as often as necessary, depending on the specific ailment. Do not allow the substance to dry. After removing a poultice, wash the area with water or herb tea.

When to use a poultice on insect bites or stings use plantain, mud, baking soda, basil, comfrey. To draw out poisons—goldenseal mixed with a small amount of oil or vitamin E, or white bread and hot milk. To help soothe and heal inflamed areas—slippery elm, mugwort, or comfrey, depending on the type of inflammations.

A fomentation is a series of alternating hot and cold compresses usually beginning and ending with a hot application.

To make a fomentation just prepare for a hot and a cold compress. Use two cloths, so the hot one doesn't heat up the cold water and vice versa.

When to use a fomentation for pains of bursitis, acute inflammations, to increase circulation and therefore activity in any area, to relieve local pain and congestion.

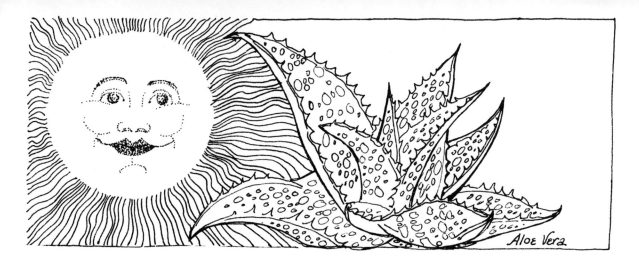

ALOE VERA:
Nature's Burn Remedy

by Rita

Aloe vera
Vulnerary, emollient, purgative

For all you people out there who may get sun-burned, or any other type of burned for that matter, I would like to tell you about an unusual plant called aloe vera.

It's a succulent of the lily family. The plant forms a cluster of leaf blades radiating from the base and growing about eighteen to twenty inches high. The thick blades contain a greenish, translucent, salve-like juice. When in bloom it bears one long stalk up through the center of the plant with clusters of greenish orange lily-like flowers. In warm climates it may bloom several times a year.

Aloe vera makes a great house plant, as it will grow with or without sun and needs little care. Keep an aloe growing in your kitchen. It's handy to grab a bit of the leaf, slice it open, and apply to a burn for wonderfully cooling relief. Aloe has also been used at my house for insect bites, cuts, and rashes. It is used commercially in suntan preparations, shampoos, soap, and lotions. Some people are capitalizing on aloe, calling it "The Magic Egyptian Plant" and selling it at exorbitant prices. You can find aloe at a reasonable price at nurseries (especially those specializing in succulent cactus). I often carry them at my herb store.

To start an aloe from a "baby," break the little plant off the parent plant carefully so as to have enough root to start. Lay the cutting out for twenty-four hours, then plant. Sandy soil is good. Be careful not to overwater, as aloe holds its own moisture and will rot if kept too wet.

(EDITOR'S NOTE: *Powdered aloe is used in many laxative preparations. It promotes the action of the lower bowel, and absorbs morbid matter in the colon, spleen, stomach, and liver. When used internally, it is usually mixed with an aromatic herb to prevent it from being constipating. It is not recommended for internal use during pregnancy, menstruation, or in cases of degenerated liver or gall bladder. Powdered aloe used externally on open wounds will absorb infected pus and help the wound close. Because of its bitter taste, aloe has been used to wean children. A piece of the leaf is rubbed on the mother's nipples. The taste is very discouraging.*)

BURDOCK:

Getting to the Roots of Good Health

Burdock   *Arctium lappa*
Aperient, alterative, diuretic

While shopping in a Japanese market a few years ago, a friend of mine picked up one of the many unusual-looking items and put it in our (straw) basket. "What's that?" I asked. "Rat's-tails," he replied. That was my introduction to "gobo" or, as we call it here, burdock.

Burdock grows in a variety of climates around the world. Gobo is a type of burdock raised by the Japanese mainly as a food. It is a strong-tasting vegetable. The flavor is that of a true root: a mixture of soil and plant. The root is collected from first-year plants in the fall or early spring. Scrubbed of its fibrous, dark outer skin, the root is fleshy and white. Some people eat it raw, but because of its strong flavor and toughness, it is usually used (moderately) in cooked dishes. I've enjoyed it steamed with carrots and onions.

As a survival food (or an addition to the homesteader's staples) burdock ranks tops. Not only the root, but seed stalks and leaves can be eaten, too. Wild burdock root will probably be tougher than the cultivated gobo, but you can find fairly tender roots of first-year plants (those having no seed stalk). Because the roots are up to about two feet long it's best to look for burdock growing in fairly soft ground.

The second-year plants are still good as food even though the root is too tough. Use the leaf or seed stalk before the plant flowers. Peel away the outer skin and eat raw or cooked.

If you decide to try burdock as a food you might also think about drying some to use later as medicine. It has long been used as a blood purifier and builder.

Skin problems, including infections, can be helped by using it internally as a tea and externally as a wash or steam. It will work on the deeper imbalances as well as the surface discomforts. It is a good addition to salves.

When fasting, at the change of seasons, or whenever you want to cleanse while strengthening, use burdock alone or in combination. A decoction of equal parts burdock and yellow dock is good. (A decoction is a tea of one tablespoon herbs for each cup water, which has been simmered at least a half hour.) Drink it throughout the day, and use it for at least a week for best results. Burdock will increase the flow of urine, while yellow dock

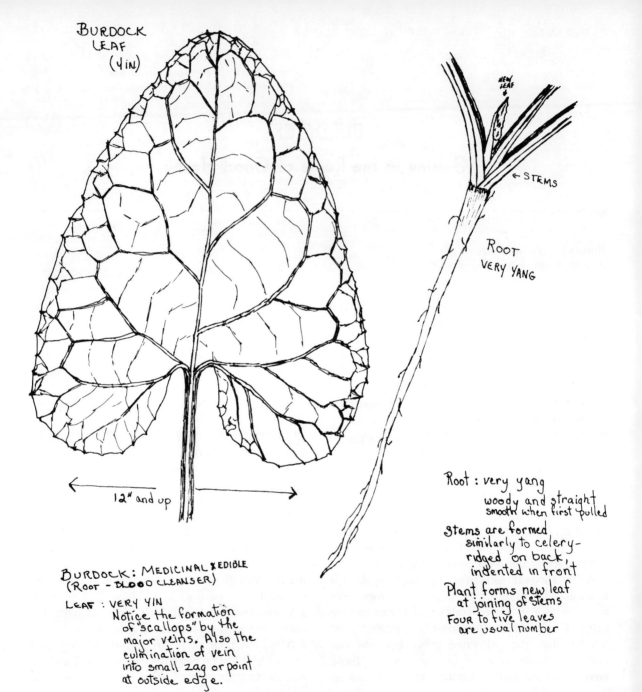

BURDOCK
LEAF
(YIN)

NEW
LEAF

← STEMS

ROOT
VERY YANG

← 12" and up →

BURDOCK: MEDICINAL ✗ EDIBLE
(ROOT - ~~BLOOD~~ CLEANSER)

LEAF : VERY YIN
   Notice the formation
   of "scallops" by the
   major veins. Also the
   culmination of vein
   into small zag or point
   at outside edge.

Root : very yang
   woody and straight
   smooth when first pulled
Stems are formed
   similarly to celery-
   ridged on back,
   indented in front
Plant forms new leaf
   at joining of stems
Four to five leaves
   are usual number

will act as a gentle, tonifying laxative. Using this type of tonic, you can sometimes fend off disease at its first signs (i.e. swollen glands, run-down feeling, minor stuffiness, etc.). Of course a nourishing diet and plenty of rest go along with this. Concentrate on working *with* the herbs.

To make a hair rinse, simmer one part burdock root and one part nettle in four parts water for about ten minutes. Add two parts vinegar and let it sit overnight. Bottle it, and use it after every shampoo.

The leaves of burdock can be used as a poultice on bruises or sprains, but the seed of burdock is unpopular with most folks. It gets carried around in socks and dogs' coats (most notably) by means of the "bur" or sticker-covered seed pod. Don't just toss these out! Dry the seeds to use as a soothing diuretic.

No wonder burdock is so potent. Its root is high in inulin, vitamin C, iron, and niacin. It can be grown from seed in almost any climate. For an obnoxious weed, it sure is useful!

REFERENCES

Hall, A. *The Wild Food Trailguide*
Kraak, Anton, N.D. *Herbs and Phytotherapy*

Although burdock usually grows in abundance where it is found, be thoughtful anyway and don't harvest more than 25 per cent of any given stash. Be sure you know what you're getting, too. Rhubarb is a close imitator, although with a good identification book or a guide, you'll find the real thing.

CAYENNE:

Hot Stuff

Cayenne   *C. frutescens,*
commonly known as red pepper

Stimulant, irritant, rubefacient, appetizer, digestive, sialagogue, antiseptic, tonic

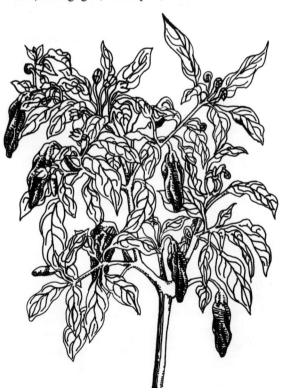

Have you ever wondered how people withstood winter before the advent of modern heating, before thermal underwear, before down jackets and decongestants? Winter wasn't any warmer then; maybe people were tougher. Perhaps part of the answer was in the use of hot stuff like cayenne. It still works today, and there are lots of ways you can try it.

For cold feet, sprinkle powdered cayenne in your socks or rub your feet with cayenne oil. Cayenne can warm you from the inside too, as any good chili eater will tell you. Use powdered cayenne in food, with other herb teas, or if you don't like the feeling of hotness in your mouth, take cayenne in capsules.

Cayenne loosens things up and moves them around. It stimulates circulation. When you want to get rid of excess mucus, cayenne will help. You can use it as a gargle, a plaster, as part of a fomentation, or again as a tea. If you enjoy hot spices, you'll especially like the gargle. (1 teaspoon cayenne, 2 tablespoons salt, 1 cup water.)

The oil of cayenne is very useful in relieving localized pain. Rubbed on a sore or cramped muscle it will bring welcomed warmth. By increasing circulation in the area, excess wastes will be removed quicker, and nutritious blood will be brought to the area. As first aid for a toothache cayenne oil relieves the pain and is antiseptic. The cavity must be cleaned out first; then you apply a few drops of oil with a wad of cotton. This won't mend the tooth, but it will sure make life easier for you.

Cayenne has many other medical uses such as stopping internal or external bleeding, in treating alcoholic gastritis, and even in healing ulcers. It is used as a tonic to the circulatory system and the liver. It is a non-toxic herb, with ill effects occurring only with misuse or overuse. It can make you feel a little nauseated at first after you take it, but that is its cleansing properties catching up with you. It's waking up your system. Practically every herbal has long lists of conditions which have been treated successfully with cayenne. It is often used in conjunction with other herbs, to help carry their properties quickly to the area they treat. Although cayenne is a stimulant, it can be used with relaxants such as lobelia for an effect somewhat like "letting go."

Although some herbalists feel confident in recommending cayenne daily as a preventive medicine, realize it is a potent herb as well as a nourishing food. Stimulating the body daily with a foreign substance, however natural and healing it may be, will take its toll eventually. Using cayenne only for a specific period of time to obtain specific results seems to be the most effective way of using it. If you are going to work on your circulatory system, really work on it—develop an exercise habit, a good dietary pattern, get into skin brushing, saunas, relaxation, or whatever you seem to need to get the results you want. When your habits of good living have become ingrained enough you won't need cayenne any more. Maybe then you'll want to work on something else.

Cayenne is so strong that it has been used to fumigate rooms, ward off attacking dogs, and do other more offensive things. It has a long history of use in many tropical cultures and civilizations. It stimulates the body's natural air-conditioning system. From the Far East to the Northwest, it's valuable hot stuff!

REFERENCES

Christopoher, John R., Dr. *School of Natural Healing.*

Griffin, La Dean. *Herbs to the Rescue.* Provo, Utah: Bi World Publishing.

Weil, Andrew. "Eating Chilles." *Journal of Psychedelic Drugs,* Vol. 8, No. 1.

CHICKWEED:
Delicious and Demulcent

by Denni McCarthy

Chickweed   *Stellaria media*
Demulcent, expectorant

Chickweed (*Stellaria media*) is one of nature's gifts that can be found all over the world. It is one of the first plants to appear in the early spring and in many places it's abundant almost all year long. I've discovered it in gardens, in moist woods, and even by doorsteps in city streets. The tender green leaves are a delicious addition to salads and can make weeding a nutritious pleasure.

Once you learn to identify chickweed you'll start seeing it often. The succulent stems are usually six to twelve inches long and trail close to the ground. The leaves are oval shaped and pointed, paired opposite each other. Tiny, white star-like flowers in the axils of the upper leaves give it the common name, starwort. Another means of identification are the small hairs that travel up one side of the stem and then start on another side at the next leaf. The leaves close toward each other at night (the outer ones having longer stems) and cover the young buds, protecting them. It almost seems as if chickweed rests at night, awakening in the light of a bright morning.

The name chickweed is derived from the fact that chickens and birds love to eat it. We love to

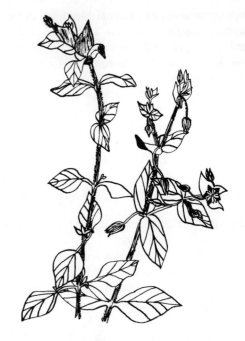

eat it too. It is high in iron, calcium, copper, and even tastes delicious. Almost every day it finds its way into our salad or juice or dressing (see recipe below). The seeds are in small capsules and easily dispersed by the wind. Once you have some in your garden you'll always have an ample supply.

Because of its demulcent properties chickweed has been used to soothe irritated or inflamed tissue. Eating it in a salad, as a tea or in juice can be healing to the entire digestive system and over a long period of time might bring some relief to colitis or ulcers. Chickweed is also helpful and building to the lungs and important in purifying and rebuilding the blood.

Externally, a soothing poultice can be made by putting the torn or chewed fresh leaves and stems on irritated or inflamed areas. If the fresh herb isn't available a strong tea can be made of the dried herb and used as a wash, or soak a cloth for a poultice. As a refrigerant it will draw impurities out of the area and will become warm, leaving the irritated area cool. Cover the poultice with a cloth or large leaf (cabbage or comfrey) and change it every few hours as needed. Chickweed is particularly good for itching from rashes, hives, measles, etc. A poultice or wash can be made and applied until relieved.

Many salves contain chickweed because it's so healing for the skin (see recipe below). Even in the seventeenth century Culpepper used chickweed as an ingredient for a salve. He wrote "Boil a handful of chickweed and a handful of red rose leaves in a quart of muscadine until a fourth part be consumed, then put to them a pint of oil of trotters or sheep's feet . . ." He also spoke of it as ". . . a fine soft pleasing herb under the dominion of the Moon." Legend tells us that it was an old wives' remedy for obesity; certainly eating a lot of greens is anybody's cure for obesity.

So start looking for chickweed on your walks and in your garden. It's a weed you'll want to cultivate and encourage.

CHICKWEED SALVE

chickweed
comfrey
mallow   } Optional
calendula flowers   }
olive oil or other vegetable oil
beeswax

Collect herbs when in their prime on a clear day; gather several large handfuls of each herb. Put the herbs through a grinder, Champion-type juicer, or tear into small pieces. Put the macerated herbs into a pot and cover by ½ to 1 inch with oil. Turn oven onto warm and leave it overnight. The next day strain through a sieve with a cheesecloth in it, squeezing out the chlorophyll-rich green oil. Add approximately 2 ounces beeswax for every 8 ounces oil and heat very gently in a double boiler until the wax is melted. Pour into sterile bottles and label.

CHICKWEED SALAD DRESSING

1 large handful chickweed
2 cloves garlic
1 cup oil
juice of 1 lemon
kelp and dulse powder
Dr. Bronner's or Soy Sauce
cayenne

Mix all the above together in the blender; add more seasoning, oil, or lemon to taste.

Denni McCarthy teaches herb classes and gives herb walks in Bolinas, California. She uses native plants for dyeing, decorating, and cosmetics as well as for her family's health and food.

COMFREY:
Super Plant of the Kitchen and Garden

Comfrey comfort
soothes and heals
builds and cleans
makes healthy meals

Comfrey   *Symphytum officinale* or *Symphytum perigrinum,*
common names comfrey, gum plant, healing herb, blackwort, bruisewort, knitback,
  slippery elm

Demulcent, emollient, vulnerary, astringent, nutritive, tonic, expectorant

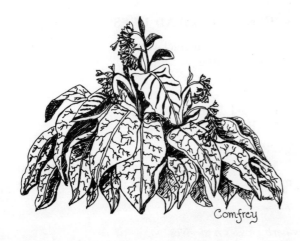

Comfrey

Have you ever *felt* an herb healing you? Fresh comfrey leaf is an herb you can actually feel working on external wounds. On bruises, swellings, cuts, burns, poison oak, bites, etc., it has done wonders. Its "magic" is largely due to allantoin, which reduces swelling around the wounded area and promotes cell regeneration. Chlorophyll, which is in the leaves, is the plant's blood. It brings the healing properties to the wounded area, like getting a transfusion from Mother Nature.

AS FOOD OR FEED

Comfrey leaf tea is pleasant tasting (quite "tea"-ish) and can be taken daily as a nutritive tonic. It is said to aid in the use of calcium in the body and in keeping the lungs healthy. It can be taken by young and old alike.

Comfrey could perhaps be one of the more important food crops of the future. It rivals the soybean in protein content and completeness (its only drawback being that it is less versatile). It is the only known plant source (other than miso) for vitamin B_{12}, which is so essential in non-meat diets. It is mainly grown as fodder for animals, its medicinal qualities adding extra benefits to their diet. Although humans can't really eat enough raw greens to rely on comfrey as the sole source of protein or B_{12}, we can enjoy comfrey raw or gently wilted (not cooked). Its flavor resembles spinach. Temperatures above 125° F. destroy the B_{12}, so if you want to "cook" comfrey, gently heat it in a small amount of water. Comfrey's prickly, tickly hairs (which are quite noticeable when it is raw) are actually good for you. They act as scrubbers internally or externally. As they might irritate some wounds, it is usually best to apply comfrey leaf poultice over a piece of muslin laid on the wound.

USING COMFREY ROOT

Comfrey root is highly mucilaginous. Its regeneration properties make it a valuable addition to cosmetic preparations and baths. It is useful in cough syrups, gargles, on bites and skin irritations, as a tea for gastrointestinal inflammation, diarrhea, bloody urine, leucorrhea, lung ailments, and, last but not least, broken bones. In Europe it has long been known as knitbone due to its amazing ability to promote the healing of fractures. The leaves and/or roots are used externally, and the leaves are eaten in large amounts. I have personally known three people who have, after removing casts early from broken legs, speeded their recovery by using comfrey over the period of a few months.

IN THE GARDEN

Comfrey propagates itself by its fast-growing roots. Even small root pieces will produce new plants, demonstrating the plant's characteristic regeneration properties. Comfrey is hard to get rid of in the garden. Plan a permanent space for it leaving three to four feet between plants. A comfrey plant looks good its first year but will reach its peak of production in the third or fourth year and continue producing for another eight to ten years. Light feeding with manure, regular watering, and trimming keep it happy. It is rarely bothered by pests or disease. The leaves of comfrey added to your compost pile will activate the decomposition due to its high organic nitrogen content. It can be grown in large pots, but keep in mind that in the garden it likes to send roots down ten feet or more.

On top of this, comfrey is a beautiful plant, growing well in sun or shade, adding its richness, even visually, to your garden. It will give you more than you need of many good things.

For more detailed information on comfrey, read:

COMFREY REPORT: The Story of the World's Fastest Protein Builder by Lawrence D. Hills, published by Henry Doubleday Research Association, 20 Convent Lane, Bocking, Braintree, Essex, England.
Available through World Research Trust, 14035 North Coral Gables Drive, Phoenix, Arizona 85023

ELDER:
A Traditional Medicinal

Elder *Sambucus Canadensis*
Diaphoretic, diuretic

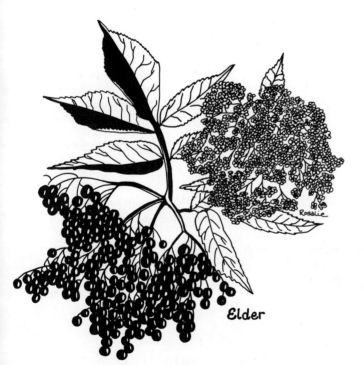

Elder

Suppose you could ask wild plants to grow in your yard. Which would you choose? High on my list would be the elder tree. Elder is common in many parts of the United States and Europe. It has for centuries been highly valued as a versatile plant. Every part has found use in the households of gypsies, peasants, and the country folks.

Collect the flowers when in full bloom to use fresh or dried. They add a delicate flavor and texture to pancakes or muffins, or can be sprinkled on salads. Although the flowers don't smell much on the tree, they develop an aroma and flavor once they are picked.

Many people have heard of elder flower tempura, but how many have actually enjoyed this wild delicacy? Cut the flowers with a few inches of stalk left on as a convenient "handle" for dipping. It's easy to collect flowers this way. To dry them just put the flower stalks in a paper bag and shake the flowers loose when they have dried.

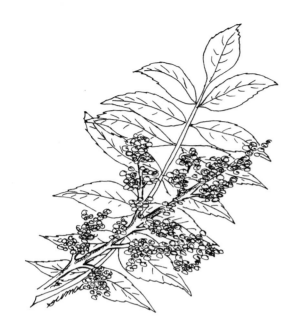

ELDER FLOWER TEMPURA

All you need is your favorite pancake batter, oil, and elder flowers still on the stem. Dip the flowers in the batter and then into the hot oil. Set the finished elder fritters on an absorbent cloth. When sufficiently cool, eat plain or dip in yoghurt and honey.

Fresh elderberries are a tempting treat, but use in moderation, especially when it's your first time eating them. Their ability to clean you out can take you by surprise. Cooked, they are less purgative, but still they retain medicinal and edible value. Add them to baked goods, jellies, or in the legendary elderberry wine. How wonderful to use food that can also be medicine. Can you imagine the delight of a sick child who is given elderberry syrup (which he normally uses on pancakes) to help his sore throat?

ELDER MEDICINE

Elderberry wine is good to have around for colds, sore throats, and coughs. The wine, taken hot before bedtime, will produce a good sweat while you sleep. The syrup is also warming and coats the throat. The fresh berries promote all types of healthy eliminations. A tea of the berries can be used in colic, diarrhea, and kidney problems to speed the natural course of disease to a healthy end. Elderberry juice is potent and should be taken in small amounts only.

Elder flowers had a place in the U.S. pharmacopoeia from 1820 to 1900 and were prescribed for colds, flu, bronchial conditions, rheumatism, stomachache, eruptive diseases, and as a blood purifier. Elder flower is a sweating herb. Blend equal parts of elder, yarrow, peppermint, and hyssop. Keep this on hand to use at the first sign of a cold.

ELDERBERRY SYRUP

Remove ripe berries from stems. Simmer in a little water, pressing out juice. Strain. Add a little ginger and cloves. Simmer gently for 1 hour, uncovered. Add honey to taste and bottle.

ELDER COSMETICS

Elder flowers are also useful for the skin. They can be used as an antiseptic wash or as part of an ointment for humans or other animals. They will ease pain and inflammation. They are an important ingredient in many natural preparations as they are softening and cooling to the skin. Think of it—cosmetics that also soothe the nerves! For a simple elder wash, put the dried flower in a muslin bag, dip in water, and scrub your face.

You can even dye your hair (or basket mate-

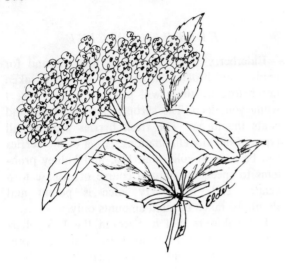

ELDER WOOD

Elder is a hard wood, but easy to hollow out and quite resilient. It has been used for making flutes, combs, spouts, bows, toys, and other items.

It is said that the cross of Jesus was hewn from elder, and also that Judas hanged himself from an elder tree. It is considered by eastern European gypsies to be a sacred tree, and its wood is not burned. Regardless of its folklore, elder doesn't burn well anyway, and is far too useful to be consumed so quickly. But then again, when you see an elder in bloom, you realize that there is something magical and sacred in its beauty. If I were a fairy it would be my first choice as a home. And if I were a homesteader, I'd try to have an elder tree around.

rials or fabrics) with the dark stain of the elderberries. M. Grieve in *A Modern Herbal* says to boil the berries in wine for a hair dye.

ELDER INSECTICIDE

An infusion of elder leaves dabbed on the skin or the fresh leaves rubbed on the skin is said to repel flies or mosquitoes. On plants a spray of a decoction of the leaves will deter aphids or caterpillars.

To keep flies off a horse, apply a strong brew of the stalks and branches.

BEWARE: There are many species of Elder. Bright red berries which taste bad may be poisonous. Do not be indiscriminate when eating wild foods.

REFERENCES

Grieve, M. *A Modern Herbal.*
Hall, A. *The Wild Food Trailguide.*
Niethammer, C. *American Indian Food and Lore.*

GINGER:

A Healing Spice

Ginger   *Zingiber officinale*
Aromatic, carminative, rubefacient, sialagogue,
  antispasmodic, diaphoretic

Nothing can compare to the sweet snappiness of ginger. Its exotic aroma brings to mind warm, balmy, tropical nights, palm trees, lush ferns, and flower-covered forests. No wonder kings of old, shivering in their cold, damp castles, paid high prices for this condiment.

It warmed them. Ginger is a diffusive stimulant. It increases the general circulation of blood, bringing warmth to cold fingers and toes. Problems stemming from or resulting in tightness, cramping, or congestion (don't we all tend to tighten up when we're cold?) are perfect for ginger.

If you want to stimulate the blood flow in a certain area externally, rub raw ginger on it. A salve or massage oil containing it is great for winter rubs.

Ginger also increases the secretion of gastric juices. It's an aid to good appetite and good digestion. (What good is one without the other?) It helps the effectiveness of other herbs used for the abdominal area. Being a carminative, it can settle a gaseous stomach quickly. The extract of ginger is so quick and sure at this that it is practically dangerous (i.e., you can soon return to eating"; when using laxative herbs such as senna, it ger is one of the best herbs for preventing "griping'; when using laxative herbs such as senna, it is a good idea to add a little ginger to ease the action.

Ginger is also astringent (touch your tongue to a slice of the fresh root and feel). This astringent property is helpful in toning female tissues, especially after childbirth. It is a gentle diaphoretic when taken hot. Ginger can also bring on a late period if its lateness is due to a cold.

Try a cup of ginger tea with honey. Or with lemon and honey it's a perfect "lemon warmer."

The highest quality ginger comes from Jamaica or India but it is grown commercially in many tropical areas. It is a beautiful plant that will grow well in a container or in the ground. It loves the sun, doesn't need much water, but can't stand a frost. It spreads by its roots, sending up new shoots as it grows. The roots can be harvested by thinning the patch once it's established.

AT THE FIRST SIGN OF A COLD

Steep:
   1 teaspoon powdered ginger
in
   1 cup boiling water
for 10 minutes.

TO AID DIGESTION

Steep ¼ teaspoon in 1 cup boiling water. Add a squeeze of lemon. Drink 15 minutes before meals.

FOR A HEADACHE

   1 tablespoon rosemary
   1 teaspoon powdered ginger
   2 cups boiling water
Steep 10 minutes. Add:
   1 teaspoon honey.

PICKLED GINGER

Slice young roots into thin pieces. Place in jar, cover with warm cider vinegar, leave overnight or longer. This is a great condiment—especially with rice dishes.

GOTU KOLA:
Herbal Brain Food

interview by David Copperfield

Gotu Kola   *Centella asiatica,* also sometimes
   listed as *Hydrocotyle asiatica minor*
Tonic, nutritive, stimulant

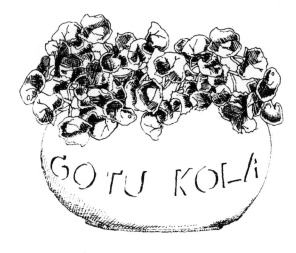

I've been interested in this "energy plant" for
about three years now. I've had some invigorating experiences and believe it to be well worth
our attention and efforts to grow it. We have a
good quantity of live plants and are beginning to
use and study gotu kola more and more. We got
the original starts from Jerry at Home Grown
Produce in Escondido. Jerry has studied aquatic
plants and gotu kola in particular for some time,
so we decided to interview him for our report to
you on gotu kola.

D: How did you get involved with gotu kola?
J: A friend of mine had a health store and
old "Doc" Stimson used to come in. He was
about ninety-five at the time and very sharp,
quick witted, and was farming a half acre. Doc
Stimson was just going around turning everybody
on to gotu kola. He gave us a bunch of plants
which we grew in a greenhouse we had.

D: Where does gotu kola come from?
J: Mostly from the rain forest floors and river
beds in Ceylon, India. It's an aquatic plant. If you
look at the plant there is a potato-like tuber which
is its main growth root. It's an exact duplicate of
tubers found on the water lily; the leaf is the
same, too.

Gotu kola is probably a shoreline water lily
evolving onto the land or maybe a land plant
evolving back to water. I don't know which way

it is going. The rivers it grows along have very soft and acid water. Also it is the mainstay food of the elephant, and according to the Ceylonese no elephant has been known to die a natural death.

D: Have you read any studies on how the plant functions?

J: That is the most fun part about gotu kola, explaining how it works. Again, it is native to a rain forest floor which is a very humid climate. The water has a lot of minerals in it, yet not *too* many; it's not overabundant in heavy calciums, alkalies, and salts like our water is here. There are lots of leaves and fish droppings from the abundant growth of life in and near the rivers. This turns the soil to a kind of peaty base that is really acid. It might get as low as 5 or 6 on an acidity scale. *Acidity puts chemicals in a liquid state as opposed to alkalinity, which solidifies things and puts them in a hardened state.* In our pipes around here you'll find crustated matter like calcium deposits because of the alkalinity. Acid state is just the opposite. You have lots of flowing minerals. Gotu kola, being an aquatic plant, drinks water; for such plants water is the only source of life. *It grows on the edge of the river with its feet or roots in the water and its leaf out of the water.* It drops its flower on the water level and the leaf takes what comes up from the roots, which is really thick, mineral-laden, acid water. It flows that water up into the leaf. In a humid climate there is rapid evaporation and gotu kola gives off water rapidly and knows that it can get more. But it does not give off the minerals, only the H_2O, *so the leaves are loaded with thick, heavy supplies of readily available minerals.* The resins in the leaf that are left behind are very concentrated minerals, more so than in any other plant that I have ever known.

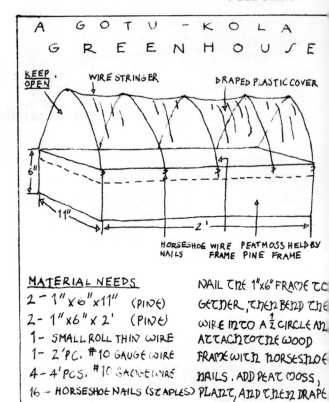

A GOTU-KOLA GREENHOUSE

KEEP OPEN — WIRE STRINGER — DRAPED PLASTIC COVER

HORSESHOE NAILS WIRE FRAME PEATMOSS HELD BY PINE FRAME

MATERIAL NEEDS
2 – 1" x 6" x 11" (PINE)
2 – 1" x 6" x 2' (PINE)
1 – SMALL ROLL THIN WIRE
1 – 2'PC. #10 GAUGE WIRE
4 – 4' PCS. #10 GAUGE WIRE
16 – HORSESHOE NAILS (STAPLES)
1 – PC. 4' x 4' POLYETHYLENE OR, CLEAR SHOWER CURTAIN
OPTIONAL
1 – 1" x 12" x 2' BOTTOM FOR KEEPING INSIDE

NAIL THE 1"x6" FRAME TOGETHER, THEN BEND THE WIRE INTO A $\frac{1}{2}$ CIRCLE AND ATTACH TO THE WOOD FRAME WITH HORSESHOE NAILS. ADD PEAT MOSS, PLANT, AND THEN DRAPE PLASTIC OVER. THIS CAN BE MADE WITH AN OLD PRODUCE BOX, COAT HANGERS, AND AN OLD SHOWER CURTAIN.

There are few plants that have the growing conditions of gotu kola. Watercress is similar but it grows in a colder climate with colder water, so its evaporation rate is slower and the minerals less abundant.

Research on gotu kola has shown some interesting things about the minerals in solution in the leaves. It has four acids found in no other plant on earth. One of them is a skin regenerator, which has been called vitamin X. The second is a brain regenerator, not just a brain food. The third is a fertility acid; it actually makes people more fertile. Just like ginseng, it stimulates the endocrine gland system. The fourth acid encourages general energy. Now I have only read abstracts of the actual studies. I read these at U. C. Riverside. They are very extensive studies. Gotu kola is a plant that has been well studied. The Herbal Institute in London brought a whole shipload of gotu kola from India just to study it. So they have lots of material published on it.

D: Can you tell us more about how the body works with gotu kola?

J: The human body is in need of minerals. By eating about two leaves of gotu kola a day, a person is taking in a high concentration of minerals. The fact that the minerals are in an acid state makes them very readily soluble. When it goes into your body it is quickly absorbed into the blood stream and deposited in various parts of the body. I understand that the brain eats last. When the body has enough minerals then the brain gets what it needs. As a person eats gotu kola the body soon has its quota of minerals and the brain begins to actually "sparkle." Just as the minerals in borage make you happy, the minerals in gotu kola can keep the brain from thinking negative, resentful, worrisome thoughts.

Normally people don't get enough minerals to really feed their brains, but gotu kola feeds it.

Then they start being able to be happy and together. They start being able to use their brains again; there is food enough for it. The body dies mostly because the brain dies, so if you take gotu kola or its equivalent in minerals, you're naturally going to live longer. The Ceylonese say that two leaves a day will add fifty years to your life. Li Chung Yun, a Chinese herbalist, lived from 1677 to 1933, that is 256 years. His diet was vegetarian, he never ate anything grown below the ground except ginseng, he drank gotu kola tea, and ate the leaves as part of his diet. The Chinese government documented his age. We've sold gotu kola to a lot of people and everything I've mentioned holds true in our experience with the plant. It is a slow reaction; you don't get a tremendous response immediately from it like you do from a lot of things, but it does everything that its herbal history claims.

(EDITOR'S NOTE: *Gotu kola is good for weak or sluggish people.* It should not be used by pregnant women or by overly nervous people. *It is a heart stimulant, but it does not raise the blood pressure. It can be used to rebuild the body, especially the brain, and remove chemical deposits, including those of drugs.*)

Jerry no longer sells gotu kola, but plants are available from Taylor's Garden, Inc., 1535 Lone Oak Road, Vista, California 92083. Send 50¢ for a complete catalog.

HYSSOP:
The Gentle Purifier

Hyssop *hyssopus officinalis*
Aromatic, carminative, tonic, aperient, expectorant, anthelmintic, diaphoretic, stimulant

"Purge me with hyssop and I shall be clean." So says the Bible. The biblical hyssop may not be the plant we know as hyssop today, but whatever the historical facts are, *Hyssopus officinalis* is a good cleanser and tonic. One practitioner recommends a three-day fast during which one drinks a gallon of hyssop tea daily. This is said to purge internal infections. Penicillin mold grows on hyssop leaves and many people use it instead of an antibiotic. Drinking hyssop tea before every meal has been found very useful in ridding the body of internal worms.

Hyssop is useful in chest and throat congestions, fevers, and colds. It loosens phlegm and has a tonic effect on the mucous membranes of the respiratory and gastrointestinal systems. A good gargle for sore throat is a tea of hyssop and white sage. Hyssop increases circulation, promotes perspiration, and is slightly laxative. For these reasons it is useful in fevered conditions.

For old and young alike it is a useful herb. The elderly use it for rheumatism as a tea and a bath. It is excellent for a weakened system. It tastes good and is gentle yet thorough.

Externally as a poultice hyssop will help heal an open wound and will relieve the pain and discoloration of bruises. As a wash it is soothing to burns, skin irritations, and sore or inflamed eyes. The volatile oil of hyssop is said to kill lice, and is widely used in colognes and liqueurs because of its pleasant fragrance.

IN THE GARDEN

All that, and it is easy to grow too! Hyssop grows well from seeds, it is a perennial, will survive hard cold winters, and will keep increasing its yield and potency for up to ten years. In Hungary and Russia where it is grown commercially for medicines and cologne oils, an acre of hyssop will yield from 1,500 to 3,000 pounds of dried herbs per season from the second year on. It is collected just before flowering.

Hyssop deters cabbage moth and is also a good companion to grapes. Keep it away from radishes though. Bees like it. It blooms from June to October and helps produce very tasty honey. A warm spot in the garden with soil that is well prepared, light, dry, but not too fertile is what hyssop likes. Have you a spare spot for this healer? Hyssop will bless your garden and your health.

MULLEIN:
Velvet and Soothing

by Elizabeth Spas

Mullein   *Verbascum thapsus*
Anodyne, expectorant, pectoral, demulcent

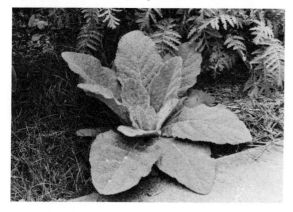

Anyone who has learned to recognize a wild plant, whether flower, tree, shrub, or herb, has experienced a special kind of satisfaction. Each day most of us pass by several species of growing things, yet few of us can name them all. Many of the plants we see and shrug off as "weeds" have interesting and valuable uses as food and medicine. One of these, quite common throughout Montana, in fact a common roadside herb to all America, is mullein (also known as velvet dock, flannelleaf, lungwort, candlewick plant, and Jacob's-staff, to name a few).

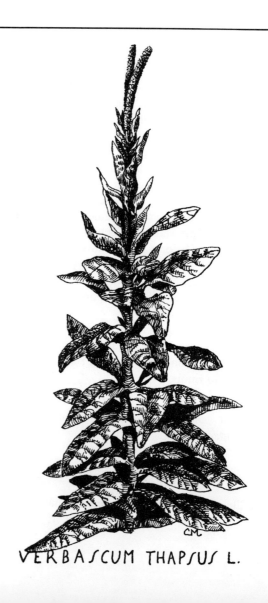

VERBASCUM THAPSUS L.

Mullein, a member of the figwort family, is a biennial plant, meaning that it does not bloom until the second season after the seed is sown. The shoot of most biennials takes the form of a low ring of leaves, called a rosette, the first season. The mullein rosette is composed of rather large, light green leaves, often 10–20 inches long, 3–6 inches wide. They feel soft and velvety, covered with fine, silvery hairs, and remain alive and can be gathered all winter. During the second season, a straight, stout, woolly, and unbranched flower stalk grows from the center of the rosette. It will grow to heights of 4–8 feet. This stalk bears leaves which are alternate, stemless, oblong, and rough on both sides. The basal leaves are large and numerous. The leaves decrease in size and number farther up the stalk, ending at the thick flower spike, usually 9–12 inches long and packed with flowers. This spike is sometimes branched, usually solitary. The flowers are light yellow and open a few at a time in an irregular pattern. They are small, an inch in diameter, with five petals which form a short tube at their base, enclosed in a fuzzy five-parted calyx. A smaller species of mullein is less thick with smoother leaves and yellow, white, or pink flowers. It is known as moth mullein.

Mullein grows in pastures, recent fields, dry waste places, and along roadsides. I gathered my winter supply along the road that runs from Hebgen Lake to Ennis, Montana.

(EDITOR'S NOTE: *In Montana this may be O.K., but generally beware of roadsides, as they are polluted.*)

MULLEIN AS MEDICINE

Mullein's medicinal properties have been known to people for centuries, and there are several legends attributing magical properties to the herb. Homer writes that Odysseus carried mullein when he confronted the enchanting powers of Circe, after she turned his companions into swine with a magic herb of her own.

Mullein has several more realistic and proven uses. The fresh or dried leaves and flowers have a faintly bitter odor and taste. The flowers contain potassium and calcium, and the leaves magnesium and sulphur. An infusion of the fresh or dried leaves and flowers will alleviate bronchial complaints, coughs due to colds, and lung troubles. Mullein tea is an antispasmodic, a demulcent, and an anodyne, especially for relief of hemorrhoidal pain.

GATHERING MULLEIN

Mullein should be gathered after flowers have bloomed, although leaves found growing under the snow can also be used. I have found Montana mullein blooming from July to October. Prepare for drying by washing carefully and tying the plants together at the base with string or rope. Hang upside down in a dry cool place, unexposed to sunlight. The herb will dry in two to three weeks. Crumble the best leaves and flowers and store in a glass or ceramic container.

PREPARING TEA

To make mullein tea, boil 1½ cups of water and pour over 1½ teaspoons of the dried herb, or 3 teaspoons of the fresh. Steep 3–6 minutes, strain, and drink cold or hot. Use a very fine metal strainer or a piece of cheesecloth to remove all of the tiny, scratchy leaf hairs. Another infusion can be made by simmering ¼ cup of the dried leaves in 2 cups of milk for 8–10 minutes.

Strain and serve warm, with honey if you wish. This milk infusion is reportedly an effective treatment of diarrhea.

To relieve head congestion caused by colds or sinusitis, pour 3–4 cups of boiling water over a cup of mullein leaves and flowers. Place your head carefully over the steam and breathe deeply.

Dried mullein leaves are also smoked in an ordinary pipe to relieve coughs.

(EDITOR'S NOTE: *Smoke of this kind is to be taken as medicine, not as a daily habit. It is thought by many that smoking of any type has its drawbacks over a long period of time.*)

Mullein has several other uses: as a dye, in cosmetics, and as a local application for external irritations. An ambitious reader of herbals could certainly add to this list.

As more people gain awareness of the serious side effects of so many "miracle drugs," perhaps we will grow more educated in herbal healing methods. The many "weeds" like mullein adorning our countryside will regain their lost respect.

MYRRH:

An Ancient Healer

Myrrh   *Commiphora myrrha*
Antiseptic, astringent, stomachic

The myrrh tree grows in the area of the Red Sea. The tree produces a glandular secretion which flows from natural fissures in the bark of the tree. This secretion is a yellow liquid which when collected and dried forms a reddish-brown resin. This gum myrrh resin is what is used for medicine and the making of incense. Myrrh grows like a shrub, rarely reaching a height of more than ten feet. Myrrh has been used in recorded history as far back as the Egyptians, who used the resin for medicine and as a preservative. Myrrh has been used for the making of incense and as an ingredient in the holy oils of the Jews.

MEDICINAL USES (MOST COMMON):

astringent, tonic, stimulant, antiseptic, expectorant, emmenagogue, vaginal douche
Myrrh acts as a stimulant to the stomach and brings about proper elimination functions of the mucous membranes in the bronchial tubes acting as a disinfectant on these tissues. Myrrh is an excellent stimulant, disinfectant, and antiseptic to open ulcerated surfaces. It lessens the possibility of inflammation and accelerates the healing action.

MYRRH AND GOLDENSEAL ANTISEPTIC TINCTURE

1 ounce myrrh powder
1 ounce goldenseal root powder
1 pint alcohol (Vodka, Everclear)
1 green, brown, or blue bottle and cork

Mix together the herbs, place in the bottle, and put into the sun; shake at least once every day. After 21–30 days strain and store in a colored bottle.
Dosage: internally: 1 teaspoon 3 times a day. Externally: as often as needed, applied to bandage and kept wet.
Uses: apply directly to fresh cuts, old sores, boils (has the properties of penetrating deeply, thus quickens healing). Use after cutting the umbilical cord. Dilute and apply to sores of the mouth and throat, or soft gums; take internally for mucus in the bronchial tubes.

TONIC

1 teaspoon myrrh
1 teaspoon goldenseal
¼ teaspoon ginger (optional—cayenne)

Add to 1 pint boiling water, remove from heat and cover tightly; steep for 15 minutes.

Uses: stomach tonic, bad breath, lungs and chest congestion, asthma, cough, general debility, conditions of excess mucus; also can be combined with a small amount of the tincture.

Dosage: 1 teaspoon every 2 hours (may be drunk in a cup of water). As a vaginal douche for leucorrhea use twice the proportion of herbs.

TOOTH POWDER

½ ounce myrrh
½ ounce goldenseal
½ ounce charcoal, soft wood ash, or vegetable ash

Uses: soft, spongy gums, pyorrhea,

CAUTION: large doses (1 tablespoon or more per day) of goldenseal should not be used by people who are known to have stomach ulcers, as the goldenseal acts as an irritant and can cause ulcers to become inflamed and bleed. Also, large repeated doses of goldenseal may cause miscarriage.

PLANTAIN:
Nature's Band-Aid at Your Feet

Plantain   *Plantago species*
Astringent, demulcent, expectorant, hemostatic

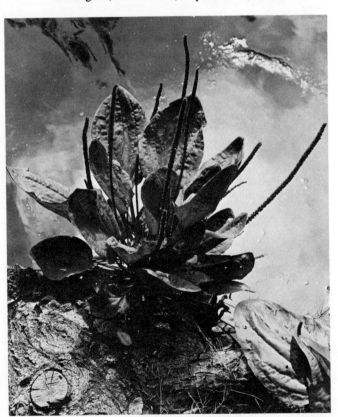

Plantain is so common that it sometimes goes unnoticed as a healing herb. It has been used around the world for a wide variety of internal and external treatments.

If you get a bee sting while playing in a park or on your lawn, look around for some plantain. Chew a leaf just enough to "bruise" it, or release its juices, then apply this "poultice" to your bee sting (or nettle sting, cut, burn, or other skin irritation). Plantain has antiseptic and astringent properties that will cool, comfort, and help heal your wounds. Plantain used externally will help stop bleeding and makes a good protective first-aid bandage in the woods. If using it over a longer period of time, change the bandage daily or more often as needed to receive fresh assistance. Keep the poultice moist. For large areas of skin irritation, make a tea of plantain and wash with it. A few drops in the eyes or a simple poultice over the eyes will alleviate inflammation and irritation from strain or smog (for use in the eyes, make the tea in distilled water, and make sure it is strained well). Use plantain in making healing salves and ointments. Don't overlook it for its commonness.

INTERNAL USES

Dry the young, tender plantain leaves to keep on your herb shelf for use in congestion of the head, lungs, or throat. Plantain loosens congestion, and it is a diuretic: it increases the elimination of water from the body. Both of these properties have their use in cleansing the body of excess mucus. Plantain is also an alterative. When used daily over a period of time, plantain tea will gradually upgrade the blood by cleansing the lymph glands and improving assimilation and elimination. Although plantain is useful to stop external bleeding, it is not used for internal hemorrhaging. It will, however, slow down too much bleeding during menstruation. Of course the cause of this should be checked into. It is useful as a douche for leucorrhea. A rectal injection will soothe and stop bleeding of hemorrhoids.

To stop diarrhea drink a strong cup of plantain tea four or five times a day. This won't constipate, but will tighten up the bowels. (Diarrhea is a good cleansing but it can be quite weakening —there may be reason to stop it.)

If none of these things is bothering you, but you have a toothache, chew on the root of plantain for temporary relief.

HELP FOR TREES

Blight on fruit trees can be treated with hoary plantain, *Plantago media*. Rub the leaves onto the affected area for speedy results.

VARIETIES

The most commonly found varieties of plantain are broad leaved, *Plantago major*, and ribwort, *Plantago lancelota*. The fruit called "plantain" is no relation to the herb.

EATING PLANTAIN

Add the young tender leaves of plantain to your salads or use as a pot herb. The green seed heads are also a crunchy, nutritious addition to salads. The seeds, when mature, can be eaten raw or added to breads or cereals.

GROWING PLANTAIN

We transplanted two small plantain plants from our lawn to our herb garden. There they've grown to about five times their original size, and they look beautiful. Like other plants they grow close to the ground when they are continuously cut back or mowed. When given space and time, they will grow to a size that will provide you with abundant foliage to use as food and medicine.

ROSEMARY:

You Go to My Head

Rosemary *Rosmarinus officinalis*
Tonic, stimulant, emmenagogue, cephalic, astringent, aromatic

Those of us who study herbs sometimes forget the wide range of uses these plants have. Many of us became interested in herbs as an alternative to man-made chemical medicines. Of course learning how to prevent and cure disease is of great importance, but learning the use of herbs for our pleasure and comfort can be rewarding too. Rosemary helped me remember this. (When taken with sage as a tea it is said to be an excellent memory restorer.)

ROSEMARY CLEARS THE AIR

The fresh fragrance of rosemary has long been welcomed, in homes and out. A pillow stuffed with rosemary and slept upon is said to prevent bad dreams and keep one young. It is burned with juniper berries in sickrooms to disinfect and sweeten the air. It is put in warming ovens to freshen the kitchen and gently flavor food. It also repels moths when placed in closets or drawers. What a wonderful herbal alternative to sickening air fresheners and moth balls.

Rosemary has long been used in perfumes and colognes. Oil of rosemary is of course widely used for the hair. A few drops on your brush each day will help bring out highlights and prevent split ends.

As a hair rinse, rosemary tea has long been used by herb-wise brunettes. It makes a refreshing addition to bath water. Why have all that hot water in the tub and not be steeping some herbs in it for your comfort, health, and beauty? Just put a handful or two of dried rosemary in a muslin bag, tie it shut, and let it steep with you. The dried herb can also be powdered and applied to the body after a bath to make you "light and merry." Rosemary tea as a mouthwash freshens the mouth and can be helpful along with other herbs in the treatment of pyorrhea. The fresh stems and leaves charred, ground, and mixed with myrrh and orrisroot make an excellent medicinal toothpaste.

A RELIEVING CUP OF TEA

It seems as if the mouth has led us into discussing some of the more medicinal aspects of rosemary. Rosemary is a cephalic. This means it acts on the head and afflictions of the head. We've already covered the mouth and hair. And remember it is a good memory strengthener. Take it with equal parts of sage as a tea. It will also rekindle lost mental energy. It has been used in cases of insanity to help balance the mind, and along with other herbs, foods, and exercises to strengthen the eyes.

Rosemary is handy to have around in case of a nervous headache. Its fragrance takes one to lush spring fields far away from any worldly worries. Part of the reason for these effects is that it stimulates capillary circulation. In this way more blood, oxygen, and nourishment are brought to the cells and more waste matter is removed. This action also makes it helpful in treating colds, colic, congested liver, and a variety of female problems. It also helps digestion when taken one hour before meals and has long been used as a stomachic tonic.

A FRIEND FOR CABBAGES AND CARROTS

In the garden rosemary is a good companion to cabbage, carrots, and beans. It deters cabbage moth, bean beetle, and carrot fly. If you bruise yourself while gardening, it will help take away the pain if used as a poultice.

As the name *rosmaris* or *rosemarinus* implies, rosemary likes the sea. It is Mediterranean in origin and will grow as a perennial in warm climates. It will grow well but not as large and flowerful in colder areas. It is an evergreen, retaining its beauty year round. The blue flowers appear now and then throughout the year in warm climates. It grows well in flower boxes or atop walls as it loves to hang like hair. It also will make a beautiful hedge, sometimes growing up to six feet tall, perfuming the whole area. It appreciates a fairly dry, fairly sunny location with well-drained soil. Since it is constantly growing, it likes being trimmed and fed now and then. It can be trimmed quite often, in fact.

Cultivate this fine herbal friend and you'll be reaping the benefits year round, head to toe, inside and out.

SASSAFRAS:
The Root of Root Beer

by Kathi Keville

> *Sassafras officinale, also known as cinnamonwood, saloop, saxifrax, or ague tree, has long been used as an aromatic, stimulant, alterative, and diuretic. The dried root bark, which is commonly used medicinally, can also be used as a cinnamon-like spice. The leaves can be dried and powdered for use in thickening soups or stews. Try it.*

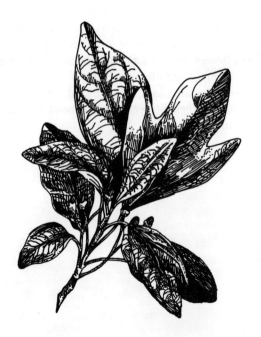

Shovel in hand, I followed my uncle up Rabbit Hill, the one I had climbed as a child. He stopped and asked, "Do you see any?" I looked around at the broad-leafed Michigan shrubbery and noticed the tree with three different leaves, sassafras. Some with oval leaves, some with "thumbs," and others tri-lobed. Anywhere from three to eight inches long, they hung thin and gracefully from the many sassafras trees that were all around us. Most of them were under six feet, but a few reached above us. Another uncle later told of sassafras trees in Georgia towering forty feet or more.

Digging was hard work, but my uncle said that the smell would keep us going. I accidentally struck one of the spongy roots and the air filled with sweet sassafras aroma. On hands and knees, we pulled away the dirt to expose brown/red-barked roots and, as we watched, the white inner bark, exposed to the air, began to oxidize and redden.

We collected, washed, and dried a number of the long and spindly roots. One whole root was selected for tea. It was soaked overnight (the traditional manner), then lightly boiled in water the next morning to make a delicious reddish tea that tasted sweet, even without honey.

It is the root bark of sassafras that is most valuable medicinally. It has long been a spring and fall tonic tea used by folks in its habitat from Canada to Florida and into Mexico. Spring and fall seem a natural time to dig it since it is difficult unless the ground is wet. It was often used with roots of sarsaparilla, licorice, burdock, and wintergreen leaves to make root beer, which, as its name implies, was fermented into an herbal beer. It was also used to flavor bitter medicines.

Sassafras is a blood purifier with its action working mainly through the organs dealing with eliminating toxins: skin and lungs, kidneys, bladder, stomach, and bowels. It is beneficial to all these. For chronic skin problems, it is used as tea and external wash, and also makes a good eyewash. It is good for digestion, particularly relieving gas, colic, and spasm. Its cleansing result is resistance to colds and infection, making it a valuable tonic during seasonal changes. It is an antidote to poisoning from tobacco and related plants such as henbane and lobelia. Sassafras will also encourage menstruation, and should be drunk only sparingly by pregnant women.

The principal active ingredient is safrole, an oil similar to that found in camphor, star anise, and cinnamon. It is yellow when fresh, and oxidizes, as the root does, to red.

The Food and Drug Administration recently banned the sale of sassafras *root* . . . yet the herb can be found for sale across the country. The FDA claims safrole, the concentrated oil of sassafras, caused cancer in test animals, so a cloud of doubt hangs over this still available herb.

Safrole is too strong to use in its pure state except externally, to remove warts. The oil can cause depression of the blood pressure and vomiting, but a person would have to drink an enormous quantity of tea to obtain an overdose. Some people (especially children) who are sensitive to sassafras' strong cleansing properties may react with a rash or nausea due to the quick release of toxins. It seems to work best when used in conjunction with sarsaparilla and other blood purifiers. An age-old Indian/folk medicine, it deserves our respect in its use, and our thanks for its great value as an herbal tea.

REFERENCES

Grieve, M. *A Modern Herbal.*
Shook, E. *Advanced Treatise on Herbology.*

SLIPPERY ELM:
Helps the Medicine Go Down

Slippery elm   *Ulmus fulva,*
common names red elm, Indian elm, moose elm, American elm

Demulcent, emollient, pectoral, diuretic, nutritive, expectorant, tonic

The inner bark of *Ulmus fulva,* or slippery elm, has many medicinal uses and has long been used for its soothing, cleansing, and nutritive qualities.

It is an excellent food for weak people, convalescents wishing to gain a little weight and strength, ulcer patients, and anyone needing a little good healthy bulk in the diet. Slippery elm feeds and soothes the mucous lining of the internal organs. It will neutralize stomach acids and absorb gastric gases. When nothing else can be eaten, yet nourishment is needed, slippery elm will provide it. In cases of prolonged diarrhea or dysentery it is quite a valuable food.

It can be used as a tea also, imparting the same qualities. It is excellent for weaning babies. It is one of the best bowel regulators for children, being gentle, painless, and tasty.

For any inflamed or irritated condition, use slippery elm in the most direct manner for quick results. In cases of bronchitis, bleeding from the lungs, or merely a tickling cough, its soothing, cleansing, and nutritive qualities are helpful. It is a pleasant gargle when combined with honey. Use slippery elm in douches, either alone or combined with other herbs.

Slippery elm has been used as an antidote for poisoning, acting like egg white in coating stomach walls to prevent damage, and absorbing the poison as it passes through the system. Pieces of the bark can be chewed for sore throat or heartburn. It should not be used by diabetics because of its high starch content.

Slippery elm tea as a wash for chapped hands or face is a blessing to the skin. After being out in harsh winter weather, give it a try.

Used in poultices on fresh wounds, boils, tumors, burns, or inflammation and irritations associated with skin diseases, slippery elm again acts directly to gently soothe, draw out poisons, and heal. Use course powdered bark for poultices and tea. Use fine powdered bark for food purposes. Gray or fawn-colored bark is best; dark or reddish bark isn't as potent. It is collected in the spring from the branches of ten-year-old trees. The inner bark is then separated from the outer bark and dried.

SLIPPERY ELM DELIGHT

This is a great-tasting food that will really tone up and clean out those old sluggish intestines.

Soak a handful of agar-agar in about 3 cups of water and heat it till it's all melted.

Add 2 tablespoons slippery elm powder

4 tablespoons chia seeds

4 tablespoons flax seeds

1 ripe banana, mashed up

handful of raisins

cinnamon (perhaps some raw carob)

Put it in the refrigerator and serve. It's like a pudding.

SLIPPERY ELM FEMALE SUPPOSITORY

Knead powdered herb with just enough pure water to form a stiff but pliable mass. Roll it into the size and shape of the middle finger. Cut it into 3 pieces (so it doesn't buckle when inserted). Place all 3 pieces in the vagina and put in a tampon to hold it all in place.

Leave it in for 2 days, then remove, douche, and repeat the whole process.

This is beneficial for inflammation and irritations of the vagina.

Keep this valuable herb on your herb shelf and remember its many uses.

SWEET WOODRUFF:
From the Forest to the Queen's Court

by Denni McCarthy

Sweet Woodruff   *Asperula odorata*
Astringent, fragrant, diuretic, vulnerary

Walking through the forest, I love to look for sweet woodruff, one of the aromatic treasures of the woods. It's known as *muge-de-bois,* or "musk of the woods," in old French. Most of its vanilla "new-mown-hay" fragrance is emitted only after drying. It is a low perennial ground cover with delicate square stems that grow from six to twelve inches long and are encircled with whorls of six to eight leaves, each having a distinct point at its tip. In late spring tiny white flowers appear under the leaves, followed by round fuzzy seed pods with little bristles that can catch on clothes or animals, and spread. Sweet woodruff is similar in appearance to cleavers (*Galium aparine*) but differs in its self-supporting stems unlike the weak and "hooked" stems of cleavers that stick to whatever they touch.

Throughout history there has been much poetry and legend written about sweet woodruff. It first appeared in literature in the thirteenth century as "woodrove," from the French "rovelle" meaning wheel, referring to its spoke-like leaves. Legend tells us that Queen Elizabeth I gave bouquets of it to her favorite subjects and that it would be strewn along the ground as the Queen passed; what a delicious way to walk! It was also dried and used in small bags to scent linen and keep away the bugs. Wreathes of it were made to freshen rooms and purify the air. In Germany it was used in May wine for a special flavor; the "Mai Bowle" is still served on May Day and the rest of the month. During the Middle Ages it would be hung in churches with roses and lavender for special saints' days. Woodruff was also used to stuff beds; such a fragrant way to sleep!

The sweetness of woodruff is due to the chemical constituent, Coumarin, which is both its perfume and a stabilizer of other fragrances. It is often used to disguise other disagreeable smells. Coumarin is also present in Tonka Beans and Melilot.

Medicinally, sweet woodruff has a tradition stemming from the Middle Ages when the fresh leaves, having astringent qualities, were used as a poultice to heal cuts and wounds. It has also been used in tea form (an infusion) as a calmative for nervous disorders, to relieve stomach discomfort, and to stimulate the liver in a jaundiced condition. Using large quantities of the herb may lead to dizziness and nausea, so use it in moderation. Gerard wrote: "It is reported to be put into wine to make a man merry and to be good for the heart and the liver, it prevaileth in wounds as Cruciata and other vulnerary wounds do."

Sweet woodruff is difficult to grow from seed, taking up to 200 days to germinate. Small rooted cuttings can be taken from the woods, a friend, or purchased from an herb supplier. (Taylor's Herb Garden, Inc., 1535 Lone Oak Road, Vista, California 92083; Nichols Garden Nursery, 1190 North Pacific Highway, Albany, Oregon 97321.) It flourishes in the moist shade and loves leaf mold soil that is slightly acid but rich in humus. Sweet woodruff can be a beautiful ground cover for a shade garden.

There are many ways to use sweet woodruff. Because of its lasting perfume, it makes a wonderful addition to potpourri. The herb can be gathered any time during its growing season, though I prefer it in the flowering stage. Collect it on a clear, dry day and hang in loose bundles upside down in a warm, shaded place until dry; store it immediately to preserve its essence or leave it hanging to perfume the air. Bags filled with the herb will scent closets, drawers, or a bath. Jars or bottles filled with woodruff will hold its healing aroma for special moments. Fresh woodruff is put in apple juice, white wine, or a sun tea (steep in a jar of water in the sun four to six hours) to extract its flavor. A pillow of woodruff alone or mixed with lavender and rose petals will make a sweet sleep. A few sprigs can be put in a letter, in a book, or given as a bouquet to a friend. I have some I gathered and pressed in a book two years ago; its fragrance still greets me every time I open it. Adding a couple of the leaves to a salad makes a nice variation. Once discovered and experienced, sweet woodruff can become an important herb in your life.

YARROW:
Stops Bleeding and Starts Sweating

Yarrow *Achillea millefolium*
Diaphoretic, astringent, tonic, stimulant, mild
   aromatic, alterative, emmenagogue, vulnerary

Yarrow reputedly acquired its specific name from Achilles who purportedly used it to allay the bleeding wounds of his soldiers. A perennial, native to Europe and North America, yarrow grows everywhere, in the grass, meadows, pastures, and by the roadside. It multiplies by its seeds and by its creeping roots.

A MEDICINAL CUP OF TEA

Yarrow tea has excellent healing properties. An infusion of it used hot and copiously will raise the heat of the body, equalize the circulation, and produce perspiration, making it one of nature's most valuable remedies for colds and fevers. It is recommended and useful in the early stages of children's colds, measles, and other eruptive diseases. It opens the pores with its relaxing action on the skin. Yarrow regulates the functions of the liver, influences secretions throughout the alimentary canal, tones the stomach and bowels, and is healing to the glandular system. It is invigorating and will greatly assist Mother Nature in removing disease and congestion from the body. Yarrow tea is also beneficial in relieving women's cramps and excessive menstrual flow, and is excellent for other forms of internal bleeding (bloody urine, nosebleed, rectal or hemorrhoidal bleeding). It can be taken internally or used as a douche for leucorrhea.

Hopefully, we won't be treating wounds similar to those Achilles treated, yet it is good to know that a yarrow poultice can be used for severe wounds and boils. A decoction of yarrow is effective as a wash for all kinds of wounds and sores, for chapped hands, and for sore nipples. A decoction of the whole plant can be used for bleeding piles, and is good for kidney disorders. Yarrow decoction is also said to be beneficial in the prevention of baldness if the head is washed in it. A caution: extended use may make the skin sensitive to light.

Yarrow has had varied uses in many parts of the world. The Cahuilla Indians used it as a mouthwash for toothache and pyorrhea. In Sweden it is called "field hop" and is used in the manufacture of beer. The Highlanders of Scotland make an ointment of the fresh herb which is good for piles. In Norway it is used as a cure of rheumatism.

YOUR GARDEN

Yarrow is easily propagated by seeds or by root divisions, and enhances the quality of oils in other herbs in the garden. Yarrow can also be sown along with lawn seed, and at first you can mow it when you mow the lawn. Let its flowers bloom in July, pick them, then mow as usual. Sow seed only in sunny places and plant by the full moon. It flowers from June to November. Gather the umbellifers in July. In the autumn dry the whole plant but do not tear up by the roots.

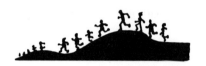

LEARNING THE WILD PLANTS

by David Copperfield

David used to be a public school educator. He enjoys devising ways of making learning easy and fun.

There are many good books out on wild edible plants. Yet I find it hard to walk through the countryside and match the plants I see with the many drawings and descriptions in books.

Now I'm using a method of learning the weeds which is working for me. I bought a spiral-bound notebook, some Scotch tape, and started going to herb and edible plant walks, nature walks, botanical gardens, and just asking friends to show me the plants they know. I usually tape one specimen to a page, leaving lots of room for notes on uses, recipes, and harvesting information. The plants dry between the pages and are easy to recognize again in the wild. I suggest leaving the 1st page for an alphabetical index, numbering the pages when you've filled the notebook. I taped two notebooks together and combined the indexes. Whenever I go on a plant walk I take this two-volume collection along, adding notes and using it as a backup for my memory.

This learning tool goes well with the *Edible and Poisonous Plants of the Western (or Eastern) States,* a deck of fifty-two cards with good color photos on one side and description, habitat, and uses on the other. They cost $4.95 and are available at natural food stores, or through Comfort Products, Box 742, Soquel, California 95073.

The other two books I usually take on walks are *Common Edible and Useful Plants of the West* by Muriel Sweet and *The Healing Power of Herbs* by May Bethel. Other excellent books are *Wild Edible Plants of the Western United States* by Donald Kirk and *Indian Herbology of North America* by Alma Hutchens. These last two books are heavier than the preceding two, but where weight is not a problem I would take the latter books.

Every time I have a chance I note information on how to spread the edible and medicinal wild plants. If everyone who picks these plants will learn to cultivate this greater garden, we will be assured of enough for everyone. Many bushes can be trimmed for up to 25 per cent of their leaves. Roots like yellow dock may be dug and the seeds spread about. By carefully pulling only the tops of chickweed and other low-growing plants the roots will survive and put out more leaves. Each plant is a little different, and conscious pickers will want to know how and when the plant propagates.

What a good feeling to become friends with more and more plants. It doesn't take long. Simply by using a notebook, your knowledge of the plant kingdom will grow like a weed.

WHY NOT PLANT AN HERB GARDEN?
A How-to-Do-It Guide

by Kathi Keville

Spring is here. Plants are unfurling, dancing, reaching for the sun, and feeling the warming earth in every root hair. It is time to garden. So why not plant an herb garden?

I've learned more about herbs from the living plants themselves than any other study could teach. When reading about or discussing an herb, it is nice to be relating to one that you have known personally. Just hearing the name will have you reflecting on the warm afternoon aroma of rosemary, or the sky-blue star flowers of borage, or the splendor of the Mexican sage in bloom.

And what more healthful herbs can you use but those grown with your own loving care? Even a window sill can provide you with your own herb garden. Herbs are easier to grow than vegetables since they are not hybrid. Naturally adapted, herbs resist predators and need little fertilizer. In fact a poor but well-drained soil and plenty of sun are what most herbs thrive in. Herbs can survive, but flourish with care.

HOW TO GARDEN EVEN WITHOUT A YARD

If you don't have a garden plot, have a garden in pots. Some herbs to grow on your window sill are: rosemary, sage, thyme, oregano, marjoram, and basil—especially if it is your kitchen window sill! That way you will keep them trimmed ·back, which will help them from becoming root bound. If you see roots trailing out of the bottom, know that they are looking for something, probably more room. Also, put a tray beneath the pot and when you water, do it until *all* the soil is moistened. If white flies appear (they'll make a telltale "cloud" as they fly about a plant) try spraying with a mild solution of water/garlic/biodegradable soap. Keep leaves from getting dusty. If they turn yellow, try more sunlight. Regular glass filters out ultraviolet sun rays, so an opened window or visit outdoors is usually appreciated by the wild-natured herbs.

To prepare a well-drained environment for a specific herb, look to where and how it grows in nature. Consider soil conditions, amounts of water and sunlight, and also temperature and humidity.

HOW'S YOUR SOIL?

A well-drained soil is one that lets water percolate down deeply. It will encourage extensive root structures that can travel easily in their search for water. Many of the classical cooking herbs come from the Mediterranean and like their soil sandy, even rocky. Some herbs will accept downright poverty in their soil. Plantain, mullein, and malva are examples of the "wasteland" herbs familiar to everyone because of their unfussiness.

Fertilizer will make herbs grow lusher and slightly less hardy. If allowed to become too pampered, though, they will not flower as fully or be as strong medicinal plants. There is a quality that comes with some struggle for existence. With the life of riches, they don't care as much to reproduce, and get lazy. There are some herbs like ginseng and goldenseal that do well on richness, so don't deny them. For any herbs, use compost, aged manure, kelp, sawdust, and other natural products. Commercial fertilizers will burn the roots. Peat moss and pine needles will create an acid soil for the pine forest plants (like buttercup and strawberry). Hardwood ashes, eggshells, and lime will turn the soil more to alkaline to please the lavender and larkspur.

Burdock, dandelion, and chicory are examples of herbal root crops. Grown in ground with rocks will make life more difficult as they grow around them. They will tend to fork in it. They'll do the same in too rich a ground where they feel life is too good. Heavy clay will stunt them, so leave that to the water-loving plants.

HOW MUCH TO WATER?

Most herbs don't need a lot of water. In fact, the essential oils will be more concentrated with less water. Little watering also results in a more drought-resistant plant and one that will not freeze as easily if it has a cold winter to live through, especially if it is not acclimated to it. On the other hand, increased water will encourage lushness. If the lower leaves begin to dry and fall, it is probably too dry. If the scent is weak and the stalks limp, chances are that you are overwatering. The better the soil is drained, the less possibility of overwatering. Most herbs hate having their "feet wet" all the time—unless they happen to be cattail, marshmallow, watercress, or other semi-aquatic plants who love the muck.

SUN AND SHADE

Sun increases oil production. It also increases chlorophyll content and greenness. Its warmth also increases growth. But if shade is the only thing you have, then especially the mints will be adaptable. Herbs grown in shade will have a more delicate flavor, so if sorrels are too sour for you, or cresses too bitter, grow them in the shade.

TEMPERATURE AND HUMIDITY

Ephedra grows in the dry high desert and sassafras in the sticky humidity of the east. Dry air herbs tend to have thick or hairy leaves to retain moisture while those growing in moist air have thin, wide leaves. I haven't had to work with keeping herbs dry, but I imagine that it is harder than keeping them in high humidity, which is done by spraying water in a plastic enclosure or greenhouse.

Temperatures play an important part in germinating seeds. Poppies and gentian require refrigeration if the winters do not freeze, and so do a few others. The seeds like sesame and coriander need warm soil or they won't even sprout. Unless you live in the tropics, vanilla orchids and clove trees will need a greenhouse. Lemon grass and vetiver and lemon verbena just won't make it through the snow. (Although this year our lemon verbena lived the winter as a dormant houseplant that lost its leaves!)

For a winter of snow, mulch well over the base of the plant. For seedlings, pull it back when they come up or they will get spindly trying to find light.

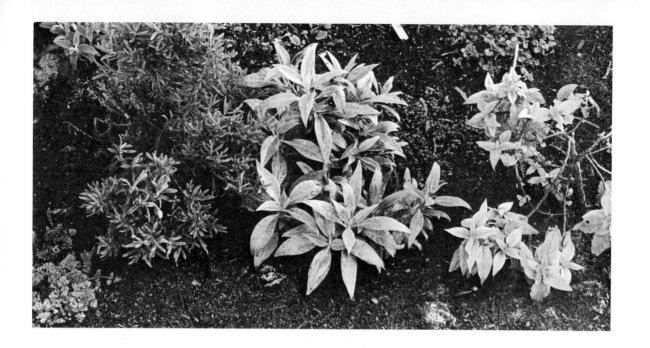

FOUR METHODS OF STARTING HERB PLANTS

SEEDS

Many herb seeds take a while to germinate. Be patient. The perennials are in less of a hurry than the shorter-lived annuals. Nature distributes her seeds lightly atop the ground from falling seed stalks. Sow them shallow, about twice the length of the seed down. Plant larger seeds in little holes or furrows and cover them over. For the light-weights, you can broadcast them (but watch out if it's really windy or there are hungry birds about). Then rake them in or blanket them with earth. If the seeds are tiny, mix with sand first for equal distribution.

Seeds need lots of water so keep them wet. If they dry out while germinating, they die. Their soil cover is important to keep them from floating away and to stay moist. If you plant in the sum-mer or fall, sow the seeds twice as deep for extra protection. If your winters freeze, herbs from such climates can be fall planted when the seeds would naturally be dropping. If you wait until the last warm spell has passed, they will soften but not sprout until the warm spring weather calls them. Then it is their choice when it is time to emerge. To avoid a too early thaw, mulch them over.

If you need to, you can seed your herbs in pots first. This is an advantage if their plot is too cold, too sunny, or planted with something else for now. It also might make it easier to keep them wet or prevent them from being trampled. They will need a special potting mix, since their envi-ronment will be so condensed. Give them excellent drainage and keep them warm to simulate Mother Earth. A good potting mixture is: 2 parts loam, 2 parts sand, and 1 part compost.

Damping-off disease can affect plants at about the "two leaf" stage. To avoid it, spread a thin layer of sand on the soil surface. Or you can use sphagnum moss for the sterile top layer. (Don't use the moss for lavender because it holds too much moisture.) Also, you can water from below by setting the pots in a pan of water which will be absorbed up.

Many herb seeds are small and will come up in thick patches so start thinning right away by pulling out the weakest and the palest. Nature makes many seeds to allow for the casualty rate. In a garden, the natural selection is not so selective. We need to help out to avoid overcrowding and competition for light, nourishment, and water. As the root structure develops, it is best to snip off the top of thinned plants rather than pulling them out and disturbing the neighbors. I've always found it hard to thin, so I sow lighter than is generally recommended. I have good results and I feel better.

CUTTINGS

Cuttings give an herb a head start because a leaf is already developed. All those stalky perennials (mints, sages, and thyme are some) are easy to propagate this way. Select a healthy stalk

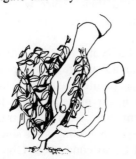

about six inches long and snip it from a strong mother plant. New growth is best. It should not be flowering, because the growth energy will be concentrated on making seed rather than root.

Remove the bottom leaves, so only a few remain, maybe six, on the top. This will help to balance the lack of roots and be less demanding on the first ones to develop. If you don't take off the leaves, they will fall off anyway, and sap the cutting in the process. Give it plenty of water but not too many nutrients so it will be encouraged to send out roots in search of them. Don't give liquid fertilizer, or it will have no need even to have roots. You can root in water, but the best medium is sand that is always kept wet. It provides a better support for the roots and doesn't encourage slime.

Have at least an inch below the cutting for roots. You can put rich soil at the very bottom for a taste surprise, but that isn't needed. Also, rooting compounds are available that the cutting can be dipped into to inspire growth, if you wish. You'll know the herb is rooted when new leaves develop. Once it seems established, be sure to feed it or transplant it so it can grow strong.

Any plant experiences some setback when being transplanted. The less that the environment is changed, the less the shock. Have the new home dug and wet. If the pots have been watered the previous day, you can usually turn the pot upside down and remove the dirt in one piece with the herb intact. Support the top dirt with the plant between your fingers and carefully slide the plant off. A gentle tap will encourage it. If the seedlings are in a flat, have enough space around each one so that they can be removed with a good section of soil.

Set the plant down into the prepared hole. Push around the soil and water right away. This will fill up any air pockets that would be uncom-

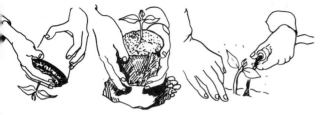

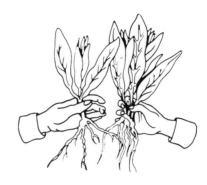

fortable. If the soil around the roots does fall off, leave the roots exposed to air and sun as very little as possible. Spread them out in the hole as you fill it in.

Plant in the early morning or evening to avoid direct sunlight until the herb is established and at home. An upside down flower pot can serve as a good shade. It can be hosed off to cool it inside if the weather is hot. Those plants with tall and spindly leaves and fine roots, anise and dill, for example, don't transplant well, especially when older.

DIVISION

Grassy herbs like lemon grass, and bulbs like irises and lilies can be divided every few years. Divide the grasses in large clumps and the bulbs individually; or you can just let them clump. Roots like comfrey and Jerusalem artichoke are so easy to grow that if any remain in the ground,

they will come up the next season. In fact, you might have to restrict them if your garden is small. When planting roots, be sure to put the top of the root up. It makes it so much easier on the plant.

LAYERING

Layering is much like doing cuttings except that the stem remains on the mother plant. This provides nourishment while it is rooting. Choose a healthy rambling stalk that will allow you to bend it gently down. After removing any leaves in that area, cover it with earth. Keep the ground watered and when new roots are established on the buried stalk, you may dig it up to transfer it, or leave it there to extend the plot.

TWO GROWING HERB GARDENS

OAK VALLEY HERB FARM: HERBS IN THE SNOW

Our farm is in the Sierras, and winter brings snow, making herb growing very seasonal.

We are in the process of developing large beds of herbs to be used in the wholesale herbal teas

and lotions that we sell. It has been a slow process, certainly not hurried along by winters of snow and summers of digging by hand. Lots of sand has been added to the clay soil. All the herbs grow in full- or half-day sun and, except for those muck lovers, don't get much water. It is a good thing that they are not used to being watered because our spring is very low due to the drought.

The annuals move around each year and are companion-planted with the vegetables. This way the beds can be redressed and the crops rotated, although it does not prevent a lot of reseeding from happening. On most of the annual herbs, we collect two thirds of the seed and store them in a not-hard-to-find cold place. Usually they are kept with their pods or stalks intact to save work. Those seeds planted in the fall always do better at knowing just when they should be coming up than those planted in the spring.

The perennials are mulched with field hay in the fall. Extra soil is put around any stalks that seem vulnerable. The herb harvesting in August and September cuts them back to prepare for the winter. I have found that retaining the woody stalks lets them decide how much to die back and will usually produce new shoots in the spring. The woolly betonies and wormwoods and sage retain their gray leaves throughout the winter, giving us a treat during warm spells of no snow. I've wondered if there was something magic in their grayness.

I am always surprised in the spring, as the leaves begin appearing through the mulch, that our herbal friends are still there. One thing nice about the winter is that by the time spring arrives, we are so anxious to garden that it is nothing but a joy.

OAK VALLEY HERB FARM is on Star Route near Camptonville, California 95922, (916) 288-3505. We have herb walks once a month in the summer and have herbal retreats.

TAYLOR'S HERB GARDEN: GROWN TO TRAVEL

Kent Taylor's family has been growing herbs now since 1947. His parents sold me my first herbs. Kent does a mail order retail/wholesale business from his home in Vista, California. The mild California climate offers him year-round growing of small plants, in four-inch pots. His main concern is for attractive and durable herb plants. They need to be able to be shipped and arrive in good shape to a store where they must wait to be bought, and then transplanted.

For shipping, Kent uses a special potting mixture that he developed. It is lightweight for traveling, and contains none of the sand commonly found in herb potting mixes. His plants are either seeded in the pot or rooted in plots of straight sand and transplanted. Then they occupy the tables and ground areas full of little pots basking in the sun and getting watered at night.

The same growing conditions are used for all herbs. That is: good soil (with a nearly neutral pH), lots of sun, and plenty of water. Kent says plants need sun, and he does have traditional shade herbs growing beautifully in full sun in Southern California! Aloe vera, pennyroyal, woodruff, and even gotu kola are doing well. They might be shorter, but Kent feels that they are hardier. He adds that his sister has the same results in Phoenix.

Kent uses chicken manure since, "A healthy plant needs food and some manure." He has sent soil samples to a service and found "organic stuff to be the best for an over-all better plant that is greener and has nicer leaves." A huge pile of eucalyptus leaves stands by his garden. "You can read a lot about bugs not bothering herbs, but they do. My new project is to use that pile of leaves for mulch and I'm wondering if that won't deter bugs."

Referring to a handsome bay tree, Kent says what a hassle bay is to germinate. It is important to have fresh seed and plant them in the dark. Don't give up, it might take four or five months!

Another touchy herb to start is angelica, whose seeds lose their vitality quickly. But Kent has kept them up to two years in the freezer. He is able to grow lemon grass, citronella, vetiver, and a bodhi tree thanks to Southern California. In general, he replaces perennials every couple of years because they get so woody with the long growing season.

To know if a plant is healthy, notice if it has spaced-out joints, is too tall or spindly, and sun-starved signs. He adds, "You can look at the plant and tell if it is happy or not."

TAYLOR'S HERB GARDEN is located at 1535 Lone Oak Drive, Vista, California 92083. Herb walks are given the first Saturday of every other month.

HOW TO CREATE HERBAL FORMULAS

by William LeSassier

This article is to explain a little more about preparation of herbs, formulas, and how to make various things with herbs. First you must realize that each plant has with it a toxic as well as remedial aspect. It also has certain elements that are neutral. Food comes closest to neutral form, but herbs swing widely and encompass a much more dramatic duality. Therefore, dosage is of the utmost importance: *the greater the quantity of an herb given, the greater are its toxic effects.* Goldenseal is a good example—30 *00* capsules a day can cause severe gastric damage, but a small dose is most tonifying. That's a very gross example.

Since every herb has a toxic, neutral, and remedial form in it we can also see that an herb may have one effect on one organ and a different effect on another. An example of this could be dandelion. Unroasted it is stabilizing to the liver and will adjust bile flow. To the stomach it is a nauseant. To the blood it's a builder (having some iron and trace elements). So you can see each herb, because it is in a gross form, has a variety of energies that it promotes. For this reason, in a given group everybody could take one herb and have fifty different responses. The person with the weak stomach could say it didn't feel right. A person with a liver disorder could say it was good. So you have another very important understanding. Some herbs are right for some but not right for others. You should be fully aware of this.

Most herb books classify herbs without giving you an indication and counterindication. They just tell you what it's good for. You should know both. Dr. Shook's *Advanced Treatise on Herbology* is one text that gives counterindications. Myrrh, for instance, is not used in some kinds of bronchitis because it increases the white blood count. It is used only if the white blood cell count is deficient. Eucalyptus will lower the white blood count and promote elimination in the lymph, whereas myrrh builds lymph. It is important to take into consideration the entire condition of the person and the entire effect of the herb. Otherwise the treatment may be ineffective. There may be many underlying causes that need treatment.

MAKING HERB FORMULAS

For this reason formulas have been created based on the laws of similar and dissimilar action. The art of combining brings about a concordance of vibration and focus. If everybody takes a formula for sweating, very likely everybody will sweat. There will always be a few who don't, but a formula makes a much more direct line of energy to the organ or system which needs energy.

The more herbs you combine, the more you need to know what you're doing. You could cancel out your formula or weaken it by adding the wrong herbs—any more than five herbs in a formula and you'd better be very good. I know many people who will read in a book twenty-five herbs for the lungs. They will often throw ten of them together. Sometimes the person will get better, sometimes not.

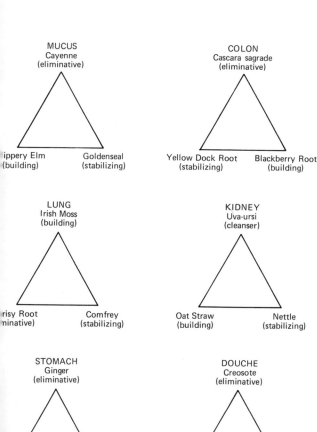

MUCUS
Cayenne
(eliminative)

lippery Elm
(building)   Goldenseal
                    (stabilizing)

COLON
Cascara sagrade
(eliminative)

Yellow Dock Root   Blackberry Root
(stabilizing)   (building)

LUNG
Irish Moss
(building)

risy Root   Comfrey
minative)   (stabilizing)

KIDNEY
Uva-ursi
(cleanser)

Oat Straw   Nettle
(building)   (stabilizing)

STOMACH
Ginger
(eliminative)

entian   Slippery Elm
bilizing)   (building)

DOUCHE
Creosote
(eliminative)

Slippery Elm   White Oak Bark
(building)   (stabilizing)

Formula making is the fine art of herbal medicine, and because each individual is different, every formula should vary in terms of content and emphasis (depending on sex, age, phase, other systems). Herbs make their mark on many subtle planes of interaction, besides what the physical body is doing. You should always ask what emotions are behind this. There are times when the emotions and mind did not cause the disturbance, but once in the body, the mind and emotions cannot help but become linked in. It's hard to believe that someone's emotions caused them parasites, or radiation poisoning. Everybody's subject to them, they are part of the general body of man. Provided these are not with the body long, they are dealt with by direct expulsion. Our emotions affect our hanging onto, or letting go of, things.

In the preparation of tea there are also levels of extraction in water: In the first 0 to 15 minutes steeped, the aromatic oils of the tea are extracted. In 15 to 35 minutes, heavier oils, some glucosides, and minerals. From 35 minutes on, minerals, glucosides, alkaloids (medicinal ingredients).

A formula encompasses the three phases necessary for each system focused upon. It must *build* the organ. It must *promote elimination*. It must balance or *stabilize* the organ. Let's look at a basic triad for the blood: yellow dock builds blood (iron rich), burdock stabilizes, echinacea eliminates. You cannot eliminate poisons from the blood without having some sufficient strength in it. Cleaning and building must go side by side, although you may want to concentrate on one action or another in terms of emphasis.

These triads are as they should be, simple and balanced. Other herbs may be added around these to form a deeper energy in surrounding systems. Just because someone gets a cold does not mean he/she has a mucus problem. That's just how it is manifesting. It may have arisen out of their stomach or perhaps their spleen. Until you learn more, you must continually question and go deeper into causes because these will remanifest in many ways.

These triads are expressed very simply and form a system of herbology called balance. Herbs throughout time have seldom been used alone.

GLOSSARY OF HERBAL TERMS

Adjuvant *aids the main ingredient in a compound to do its work.*

Alterative *herbal agents that are tonics for the blood, which gradually alter and correct an impure blood condition, restoring healthy function to the different organs without inducing perceptible bowel evacuation.*

Anodyne *herbal agents that allay or relieve pain by reducing the sensitivity of the nerves.*

Anthelmintics *herbal agents used to expel stomach and intestinal worms and herbal agents that destroy intestinal worms without necessarily causing their evacuation.*

Antiarthritics *used to relieve arthritic conditions, break up calcification, relieve locked joints, the muscles, and nerves.*

Antibilious *reduces excess secretion of bile.*

Antiemetic *used to prevent or relieve vomiting or nausea.*

Antihydropics *used to relieve dropsy, will give relief to those having difficulty voiding or evacuating urine.*

Antilithics *used to relieve calculous affections such as kidney stones, gall stones, and other concretions in the joints and muscles.*

Antiphlogistic *works against inflammation.*

Antipyretic *used to relieve body temperatures in fevers, usually by cooling internally rather than by inducing sweat.*

Antirheumatics *used to prevent, relieve, or cure rheumatism.*

Antiscorbutic *nutritional-type herb used to prevent or relieve scurvy.*

Antiseptic *inhibit the growth of micro-organisms on living tissue.*

Antispasmodics *used to prevent or ease muscular spasms or convulsions.*

Antisyphilitics *relieve or cure venereal disease.*

Aperients *mildly laxative (for babies, infants, very weak people) without purging.*

Aphrodisiac *provokes or excites sexual function or desire.*

Aromatic *characterized by fragrant smell, pungent, spicy taste. Stimulant to gastrointestinal mucous membrane. Also used to disguise strong, bitter, or unpleasant taste of herbs which are necessary to take. Aromatics can prevent griping in the bowels.*

Astringent *agents that promote greater density and firmness of tissue checking discharge of mucus and fluid from the body.*

Bitter(s) *tastes bitter and stimulates appetite and gastric secretion.*

Carminative *used to relieve colic, grippe, flatulence, or expel gas from the intestine.*

Cathartic *used to cleanse liver, gall ducts, alimentary canal; normalize peristaltic action of the bowels and accelerate a cleansing by evacuation from the bowel.*

Cephalic *useful for disorders of the head.*

Cholagogues *agents which act upon the liver, stimulating the secretion and flow of bile.*

Condiment *adds flavors to foods.*

Cordial   *strengthening to heart.*

Corrective   *used to correct or render more pleasant the action of other herbal remedies.*

Counterirritant   *used to produce superficial inflammation of the skin in order to relieve deeper inflammation.*

Demulcent   *used to soothe, soften, and allay irritation of mucous membranes.*

Deobstruent   *removes obstruction in the alimentary canal.*

Depilatory   *removes hair.*

Depurant   *cause waste elimination, purifies the body system.*

Detergent   *agent for cleansing wounds, boils, ulcers.*

Diaphoretic   *promotes moderate sweating.*

Diuretic   *increases excretion of urine by dilation or irritation.*

Emetics   *used to induce vomiting.*

Emmenagogues   *agents that promote the menstrual flow and discharge.*

Emollient   *externally softens, counteracts dry skin; internally soothes inflamed surface of mucous membranes.*

Errhine   *induces flow of mucus from nasal passages, often causes sneezing.*

Esculent   *good as a food.*

Expectorant   *used to expel mucus from respiratory tract.*

Febrifuge   *reduces or prevents fever.*

Galactagogue   *used to stimulate and promote secretion of milk.*

Hemagogue   *promotes flow of blood.*

Hemostatic   *stops bleeding from wounds.*

Hepatic   *influence liver, increase flow of bile.*

Homeostatic   *arrests bleeding and hemorrhages.*

Hydragogue   *dispels watery fluid, as from bowels.*

Irritant   *excites a characteristic action or function.*

Laxative   *loosens the bowels.*

Maturating   *produces discharge of pus, brings boils to "head."*

Narcotic   *induces unconsciousness or drowsiness.*

Nauseant   *produces nausea, or inclination to vomit.*

Nervine   *soothes or relieves disorders of nerves.*

Nutritives   *assist assimilation, nourish and build the body tissue.*

Ophthalmics   *used for diseases of the eye.*

Parturients   *used to induce labor and expel placenta.*

Pectoral   *used to treat diseases of the respiratory tract.*

Peristaltics   *used to increase peristalsis or muscular contraction in the bowels.*

Purgatives   *used only in emergencies to induce copious evacuation of the bowels.*

Refrigerants   *used to lower body temperature.*

Restorative   *helps to bring a person back to consciousness.*

Rubefacient   *causing redness of the skin due to increased blood supply; usually works by irritation (see definition of irritant).*

Sedative   *quiets or allays irritability or pain.*

Sialagogue   *used to excite salivary glands, provoke secretion, and increased flow of saliva.*

Soporific   *used to induce sleep.*

Stimulant   *quickens functional activity of tissues.*

Stomachics   *give strength and tone to the stomach. Stimulate digestion and/or appetite.*

Sudorific   *produces heavy perspiration.*

Tonic   *improves body tone by stimulating tissue nutrition; invigorates, restores, or stimulates the system.*

Vermifuge   *see anthelmintic.*

Vesicant   *causes blisters.*

Vulneraries   *healing to fresh cuts or wounds.*

INDEX

Medicine; Health

WELL-BEING

Edited by Barbara Salat
& David Copperfield

In 1975 *Well-Being* Magazine was founded in response to people's growing interest in natural health care. This book contains the best and most useful articles that have appeared in the magazine, and is full of down-to-earth, practical information on modern folk medicine and natural methods of caring for one's health. There are articles on diet, with recipes and suggestions on food preparation, on preventive home remedies and natural healing, on herb preparations and how to use them, and more. WELL-BEING is a friendly and informative "do-it-yourself" guide to healthy living, written by *modern pioneers* —back-to-the-landers, gardeners, teachers, cooks, doctors, midwives, and just plain people.

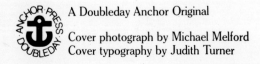

A Doubleday Anchor Original

Cover photograph by Michael Melford
Cover typography by Judith Turner

ISBN: 0-385-14221-8

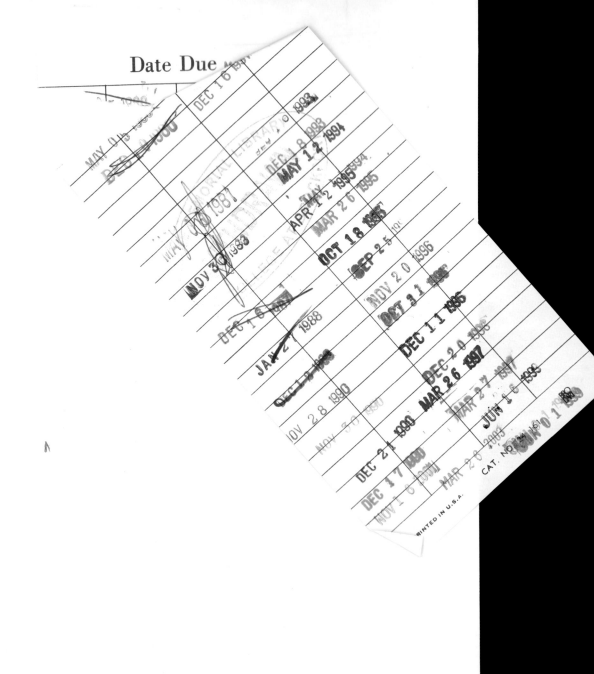

Date Due